☞ **BEFORE USING STEMI ASSISTANT IN THE CLINICAL SETTING, PLEASE REVIEW BOOK AND BECOME FAMILIAR WITH ITS CONTENT AND LAYOUT -** *this will facilitate rapid access to critical information during a STEMI Emergency.*

How to use STEMI ASSISTANT:

1. Refer to the UNIVERSAL ACS PATIENT MANAGEMENT ALGORITHM (on page 1) when caring for patients with Chest Pain or other possible symptoms of Acute Coronary Syndrome (ACS).

2. Obtain STAT 12 Lead ECG on patient suspected of suffering from ACS.

3. Evaluate the patient's 12 Lead ECG and identify any leads where abnormal ST Elevation is noted.   If you are not certain what constitutes "ST Segment Elevation," refer to diagram on back cover of book and page 9 for assistance in determining ST Segment and T wave patterns that are commonly associated with STEMI and other ACS conditions.

4. Correlate the leads where your patient has the HIGHEST DEGREE of ST Elevation with the Color-coded ECG on the FRONT COVER of this book.

5. Follow the arrow from the LEAD SET where the patient's ECG shows the highest ST Elevation to the page number listed in the arrowhead.   Open book to the indicated page.

6. If your patient's ST patterns don't match those on the ECG featured in the book, scroll forward through the book until you find an ECG where the ST segment patterns most closely resemble that of your patient's.

7. Refer to the information presented in the OPEN PAGES to assist you in the care of your patient.

Tutorial Video - go to: www.ECGtraining.org →   STEMI Assistant →   Tutorial Video

---

Table of Contents (in Universal Algorithm)	1
Abbreviations used in this book	37
Reference Sources	37
Author / Publisher information	38

STEMI Assistant

Authored by:

Wayne W Ruppert, CVT, CCCC, NREMT-P
Cardiovascular Clinical Coordinator
Bayfront Health Dade City

Editorial Board:

Barbra E. Backus, MD, PhD
Developer of The HEART Score
University Medical Center, Utrecht, Netherlands

Michael R. Gunderson,
National Director, Clinical Systems, Quality and Health I.T.
American Heart Association

Anna Ek, RN, BSN
Accreditation Specialist
The Society of Cardiovascular Patient Care

William Parker, PharmD, CGP
Director of Pharmacy Services
Bayfront Heath Dade City

Publisher Information:

TriGen Publishing Company
www.TriGenPress.com
Marketed and Distributed Worldwide by The Ingram Book Company
© copyright 2015 Wayne Ruppert
ISBN: 978-0-9829172-5-1
Library of Congress Catalog Number: PENDING

© 2015 Wayne Ruppert. All contents of this book, including but not limited to text and graphic art images have been registered with the US Patent and Trademark Office in Washington, DC. No part of this book may be reproduced and/or distributed without written consent of the author.

> COPYRIGHT EXCEPTIONS: This book may be reproduced by employees, physicians and contractors of Community Health Systems (CHS), its affiliated hospitals and associated emergency medical services (EMS) providers for educational purposes and use in the clinical setting. PDF file download information will be distributed via the following CHS networks: CHS Intranet, All Chest Pain Center Coordinators; All Emergency Department Directors and All Cath Lab Directors internal email networks. A PDF copy of this book will be available to all CHS and CHS affiliated team members. To obtain a PDF copy of this book, CHS and CHS affiliated team members should email their request to: wayne.ruppert@bayfronthealth.com from their CHS or CHS affiliated email address.

Electronic versions of this book, including an iBooks version and smartphone Apps, are currently being developed. See www.ECGtraining.org for updates Click link: STEMI Assistant.

---

*Dedicated to Gail Ruppert and Wayne W Ruppert, Sr. (5/14/1926 - 12/11/2010), whose unconditional love and guidance determined my future.
And to Jeremy Ruppert, Caitlin Cameron, Wayne W "Will" Ruppert, III, Kinsley Nicole Ruppert and Emma Adalyn Ruppert, who ARE the future*

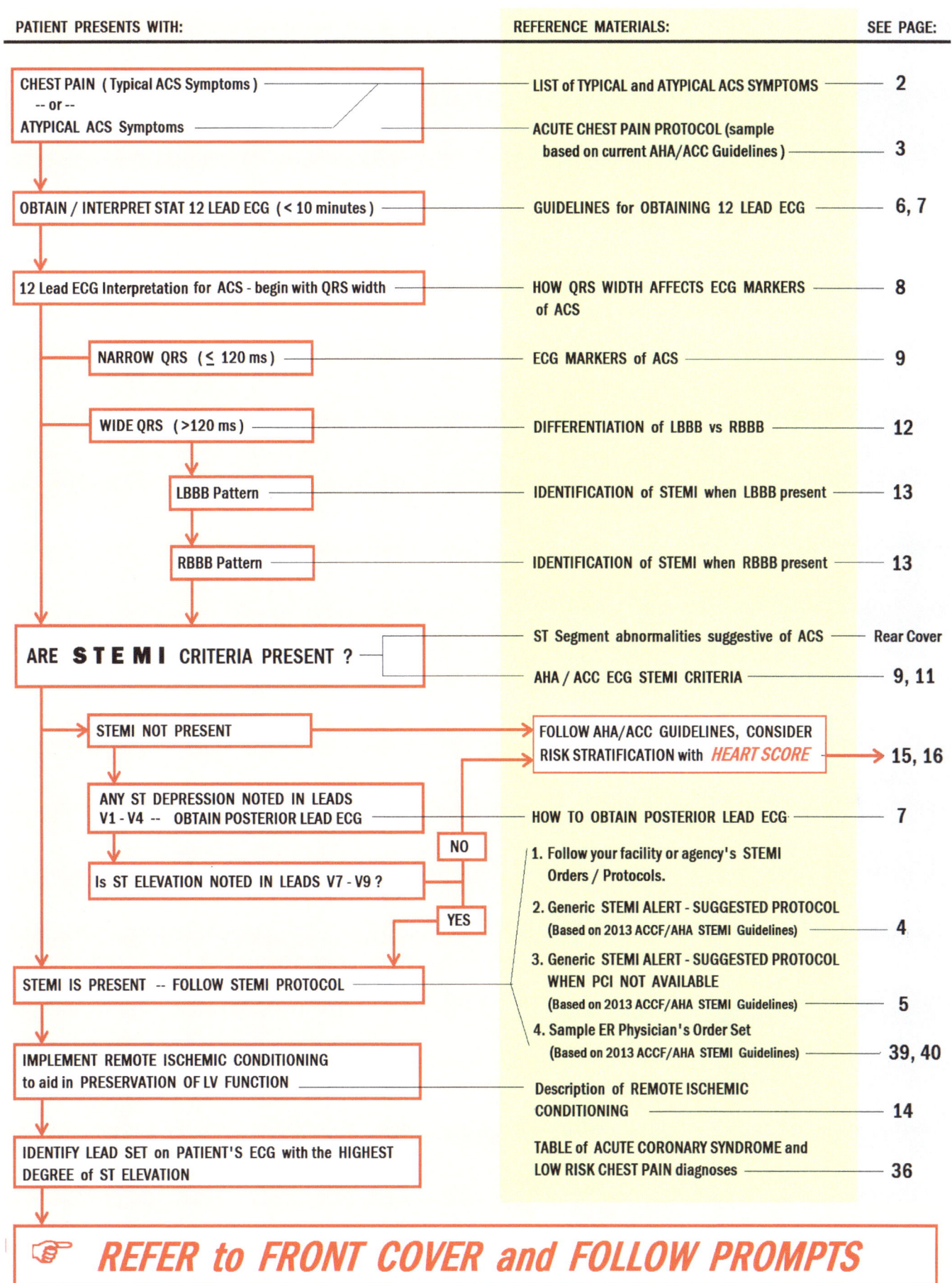

TYPICAL SYMPTOMS of ACUTE CORONARY SYNDROME:

- ☐ RETROSTERNAL CHEST PRESSURE or CHEST PAIN (often described as "dull or pressure-like" sensation).
- ☐ Chest pain may RADIATE to shoulders, neck, jaw, left and/or right arm.
- ☐ Pain is USUALLY not affected by POSITION, MOVEMENT or DEEP INSPIRATION.
- ☐ Pain may be INTERMITTENT, waxing and waning for days or weeks preceding Acute Myocardial Infarction.
- ☐ COLD SWEATS often present
- ☐ SHORTNESS of BREATH may or may not be present
- ☐ NAUSEA / VOMITING may or may not be present

ATYPICAL SYMPTOMS of ACUTE CORONARY SYNDROME (includes but not limited to):

- ☐ PAIN or PRESSURE in any area of the body where CHEST PAIN radiates to, MINUS the central chest pain: e.g.: unexplained NECK, SHOULDER, JAW (tooth) and Left and/or Right arm pain.
- ☐ ABDOMINAL PAIN / "INDIGESTION" - typically upper abdomen, mid-epigastric region
- ☐ SHORTNESS of BREATH
- ☐ NAUSEA / VOMITING
- ☐ EXTREME WEAKNESS / FATIGUE
- ☐ COLD SWEATS
- ☐ PALPITATIONS / ELEVATED HEART RATE

According to a multi-center study comprised of over 434,000 patients, the PREDISPOSING FACTORS for patients who experience ATYPICAL Symptoms of ACS include patients who are FEMALE, DIABETIC, NON-CAUCASIAN, OVER AGE 75, and have PREVIOUS HISTORIES of STROKE and/or HEART FAILURE.

The more of PREDISPOSING FACTORS for experiencing ACS without CHEST PAIN that a patient has, the higher the probability that the patient will suffer ACS without experiencing CHEST PAIN. The table below illustrates this:

The EFFECT of Having MULTIPLE PREDISPOSING FACTORS for ACUTE MI without Chest Pain

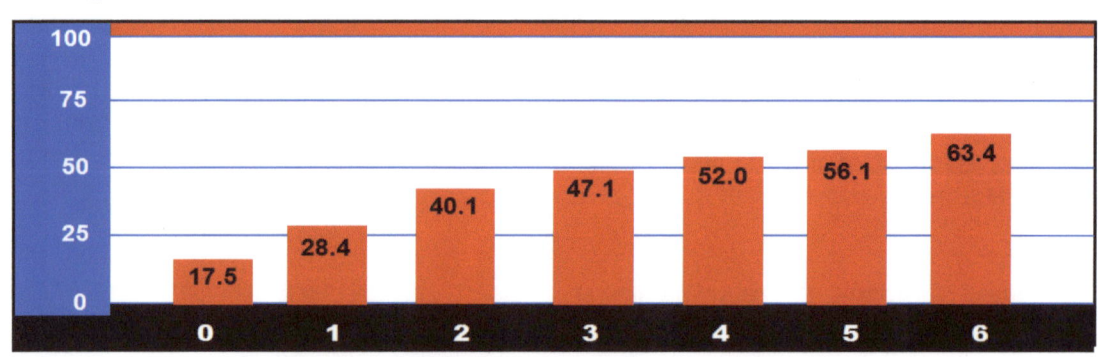

PREDISPOSING FACTORS: **S**troke (previous), **H**eart failure (previous), **R**ace (non-white), **E**lderly (age 75+), **W**omen, **D**iabtetes

DATA SOURCE: J. CANTO, MD, MSPH, et al, JAMA 2000 ; 283 : 3223 - 3229

ACUTE CHEST PAIN - SUGGESTED PROTOCOL

OUT OF HOSPITAL / NON-CLINICAL SETTING:

- ☐ Call 911 --DO NOT HANG UP (if you're alone with patient put phone on SPEAKER if possible)
- ☐ ASPIRIN 325mg (or four 81mg children's aspirin) -- have patient CHEW tablet(s)
- ☐ AED -- If available, have it ready but *DO NOT activate it unless patient becomes PULSELESS*

EMS & HOSPITAL SETTING:

- ☐ Administer oxygen only when *SAO2 is less than 92% and/or when signs of hypoxemia are present -*
    --- titrate to maintain SAO2 between 92 - 99%
- ☐ ASPIRIN 325mg (or four 81mg children's aspirin) -- have patient CHEW tablet(s)
- ☐ IV Normal Saline, preferably 20g IV catheter or larger, antecubital vein, KVO rate
- ☐ Continuous ECG Monitoring
- ☐ OBTAIN and INTERPRET 12 Lead ECG within 10 minutes of patient arrival or onset of symptoms
    - **IF STEMI is present - INITIATE STEMI ALERT.** (Refer to STEMI ALERT - SUGGESTED PROTOCOL on pages 4 & 5, and sample ER physician's order set on pages 39 & 40) Goal is to achieve FIRST MEDICAL CONTACT (FMC) - to - REPERFUSION in <90 MINUTES for ALL PATIENTS.

    EMS: in STEMI, transport to NEAREST PCI Capable Chest Pain Center - PROVIDE ADVANCED NOTIFICATION of STEMI Alert and if capable transmit 12 Lead ECG, ASAP.

- ☐ If ECG is normal in HIGH RISK, SYMPTOMATIC patient, obtain RIGHT SIDED and POSTERIOR Lead (18 Lead) ECG. (see page 7) IF ECG is normal in the HIGH RISK, SYMPTOMATIC patient, repeat ECG every 15-30 minutes for the first hour, at 3 and 6 hours, and whenever symptoms change.
- ☐ Obtain STAT Troponin, and then repeat at 3 and 6 hours. If patient exhibits on-going, suspicious symptoms obtain additional Troponin samples beyond 6 hours.
- ☐ NITROGLYCERIN 0.4 mg. sublingual tablet or spray. Re-assess patient for symptoms every 5 minutes, may repeat dose twice (3 dose total).
    NITROGLYCERIN CONTRAINDICATED if patient has:
    - Systolic BP < 90mm/hg
    - RIGHT VENTRICULAR MI -- IF INFERIIOR WALL MI is noted on 12 Lead ECG, OBTAIN RIGHT-SIDED ECG prior to administration of Nitroglycerin (see pages 28-31)
    - Taken VIAGRA in the past 24 hours
    - Taken LEVITRA in the past 24 hours
    - Taken CIALIS in the past 48 hours
- ☐ Calculate ACS Risk Stratification Score (see HEART Score page 15 & 16)
- ☐ Morphine Sulfate: 2 - 5 mg. IV every 5 - 30 minutes as needed for pain unless contraindicated / OR per protocol / physician order. Use caution in Right Ventricular MI
- ☐ BETA BLOCKER per unit protocol / physician order. CONTRAINDICATED if systolic BP < 90mm/hg
- ☐ FOLLOW ACLS GUIDELINES for DYSRHYTHMIA MANAGEMENT

Reference sources: 2013 ACCF/AHA Guidelines for Management of Patients with STEMI ; 2014 AHA/ACCF Guidelines for Management of Patients with NSTEMI / ACS

STEMI ALERT - SUGGESTED PROTOCOL:

- ☐ Reperfusion therapy is recommended for all eligible patients whose symptom onset is within 12 hours, or whose symptom onset is between 12 and 24 hours when there is clinical and/or ECG evidence of ongoing ischemia
- ☐ PRIMARY PCI within 90 minutes of First Medical Contact (FMC) is the preferred method of reperfusion.
- ☐ Immediate angiography and PCI should be performed for resuscitated out-of-hospital cardiac arrest patients whose initial ECG shows STEMI
- ☐ EMS: Transport patient to nearest PCI-Capable Chest Pain Center. IF there are no PCI-Capable facilities available to provide FMC-to-PCI within 120 minutes, transport to the nearest hospital capable of providing immediate Fibrinolytic Therapy, and follow STEMI ALERT - SUGGESTED PROTOCOL when PCI NOT AVAILABLE on page 5. Provide advanced notification of STEMI Alert and if capable, transmit 12 Lead ECG to receiving hospital as soon as possible.
- ☐ Oxygen, IV, Aspirin, Nitroglycerin and Morphine therapy as per Acute Chest Pain Protocol, page 3
- ☐ Consider REMOTE ISCHEMIC CONDITIONING when it will not delay reperfusion, and there are no contraindications (see page 14)
- ☐ P2Y12 Receptor Inhibitor Therapy should be given as early as possible or at time of primary PCI to patients with STEMI. (Class I Recommendation, L.O.E. B) Options include: Clopidogrel* (Plavix) 600mg oral; Prasugrel (Effient) 60mg oral (Prasugrel contraindicated in patients with history of stroke or TIA. Also note Prasugrel has not been studied in patients <60kg and patients >75 years of age); Ticagrelor (Brilinta) 180mg oral
- ☐ Beta Blocker therapy is indicated (Class I Recommendation, L.O.E. B) for STEMI unless any of following CONTRAINDICATIONS are PRESENT: heart failure/low output state; heart rate <60; P-R Interval > 240ms, 2nd or 3rd Degree Heart Block; active asthma; increased risk for cardiogenic shock**
- ☐ It is reasonable to consider administration of IV GP IIb/IIIa receptor agonist therapy in the PRE-Cardiac Cath setting in patients whom primary PCI is intended. (Class IIb, Recommendation, L.O.E. B)

* Two loading dose regimens for Plavix are described: 600mg and 300mg oral. According to Mehta et al (NEJM 2010;363:930-942) both dosing regimens when given with aspirin have similar incidents of major bleeding (2.5% vs. 2.0%), however the 600mg regimen group had a lower rate of post-PCI in-stent thrombus (1.6% vs. 2.3%). Many practitioners will give Plavix 300mg prior to Cardiac Cath, and give the remaining 300mg after successful PCI.

** Risk Factors for Cardiogenic Shock (the greater number of risk factors present, the higher the risk of developing Cardiogenic Shock): age >70 years, Systolic BP <120 mm/hg, sinus tach >110 bpm, heart rate <60, and increased time since onset of STEMI symptoms.

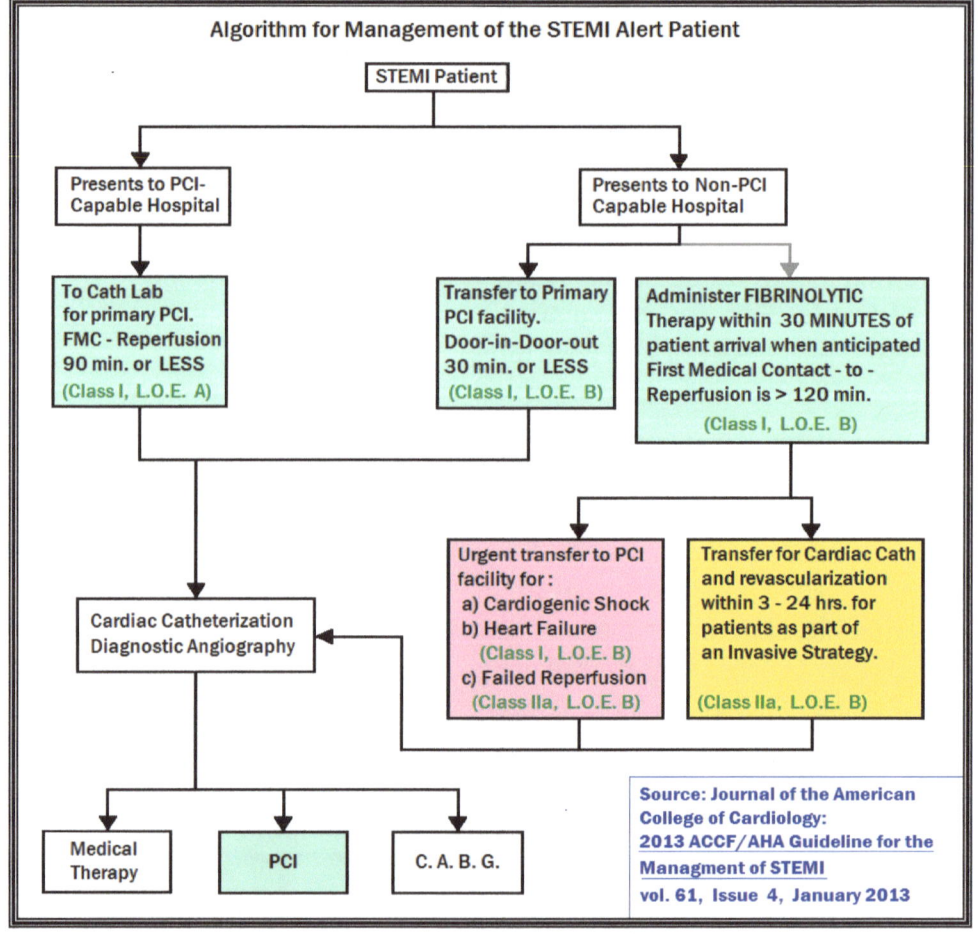

Algorithm for Management of the STEMI Alert Patient

Source: Journal of the American College of Cardiology: 2013 ACCF/AHA Guideline for the Managment of STEMI vol. 61, Issue 4, January 2013

STEMI ALERT - SUGGESTED PROTOCOL when PCI NOT AVAILABLE:

- ☐ Follow ACUTE CHEST PAIN PROTOCOL (page 3)
- ☐ If PCI Cannot be performed WITHIN 120 minutes of FMC, in the ABSENCE of CONTRAINDICATIONS, FIBRINOLYTIC THERAPY should be given to patients with STEMI when the ONSET of ischemic symptoms are within 12 hours (CLASS I Recommendation, Level of Evidence A) or when the onset of ischemic symptoms are within 12 - 24 hours and there is clinical and/or ECG evidence of ongoing ischemia and a large area of myocardium is at risk and/or hemodynamic instability is present (CLASS IIa Recommendation, Level of Evidence C).
- ☐ FIBRIN-SPECIFIC Fibrinolytic Agents are preferred over non-fibrin specific agents, and include:
    - Tenectaplase (TNK-tPA)   Single IV weight-based bolus
    - Reteplase (rPA)   10 unit + 10 unit boluses given 30 minutes apart
    - Alteplase (tPA)   90 minute weight based infusion
- ☐ ANTIPLATELET THERAPY to be given WITH Fibrinolytic Therapy includes the administration of Aspirin (162-300mg loading dose) and clopidogrel (Plavix) : 300-mg loading dose for patients 75 or less years of age; 75-mg loading dose for patients >75 years of age (Class I Recommendation, L.O.E. A)
- ☐ ANTICOAGULATION THERAPY to be given WITH Fibrinolytic Therapy include EITHER the administration of Unfractionated Heparin (UFH) OR Enoxaparin (Lovenox). (Class I Recommendation)
    - UFH dosage: 60 U/kg (maximum 4,000U) IV bolus followed by infusion of 12 U/kg/hr (maximum 1000 Units) initially, adjusted to maintain aPTT at 1.5 to 2.0 times the control value for 48 hours or until revascularization is achieved. (Class I Recommendation, L.O.E. C)
    - LOVENOX dosage: Age <75 y: 30mg IV bolus followed in 15 minutes by 1mg/kg subcutaneously every 12 hrs (max. 100mg for first 2 doses); if age 75 or more, NO bolus, 0.75mg/kg subcutaneously every 12 hrs, (max. 75mg for the first 2 doses); if Creatinine Clearance is less than 30ml/min, dosage is 1mg/kg subcutaneously every 24 hrs (all ages).
    (Class I Recommendation, L.O.E. A)
- ☐ IMMEDIATE TRANSFER of STEMI patients after Fibrinolytic therapy to a PCI-capable facility is indicated in the following circumstances: patients who develop CARDIOGENIC SHOCK and/or severe HEART FAILURE (Class I Recommendation, L.O.E B) and /or patients with evidence of FAILED reperfusion or re-occlusion AFTER Fibrinolytic therapy (Class IIa Recommendation, L.O.E. B)

ABSOLUTE CONTRAINDICATIONS TO FIBRINOLYTIC THERAPY:

- ☐ ANY prior INTRACRANIAL HEMORRHAGE; STRUCTURAL CEREBRAL LESION (e.g. Arteriovenous Malformation - AVM); MALIGNANT INTRACRANIAL NEOPLASM; ISCHEMIC STROKE within past 3 MONTHS (except Acute ISCHEMIC Stroke WITHIN 4.5 hours)
- ☐ INTRACRANIAL or INTRASPINAL SURGERY WITHIN 2 MONTHS
- ☐ SIGNIFICANT CLOSED-HEAD or FACIAL TRAUMA WITHIN 3 MONTHS
- ☐ SUSPECTED AORTIC DISSECTION
- ☐ ACTIVE BLEEDING or BLEEDING DIATHESIS (except menses)
- ☐ SEVERE, UNCONTROLLED HYPERTENSION (not responsive to emergency therapy)
- ☐ For STREPTOKINASE: Prior treatment with STREPTOKINASE within previous 6 months

NOTE: The source for ALL RECOMMENDATIONS listed on PAGES 4 and 5 are from:
2013 ACCF/AHA Guideline for the Management of STEMI.

GUIDELINES FOR OBTAINING 12 LEAD ECG:

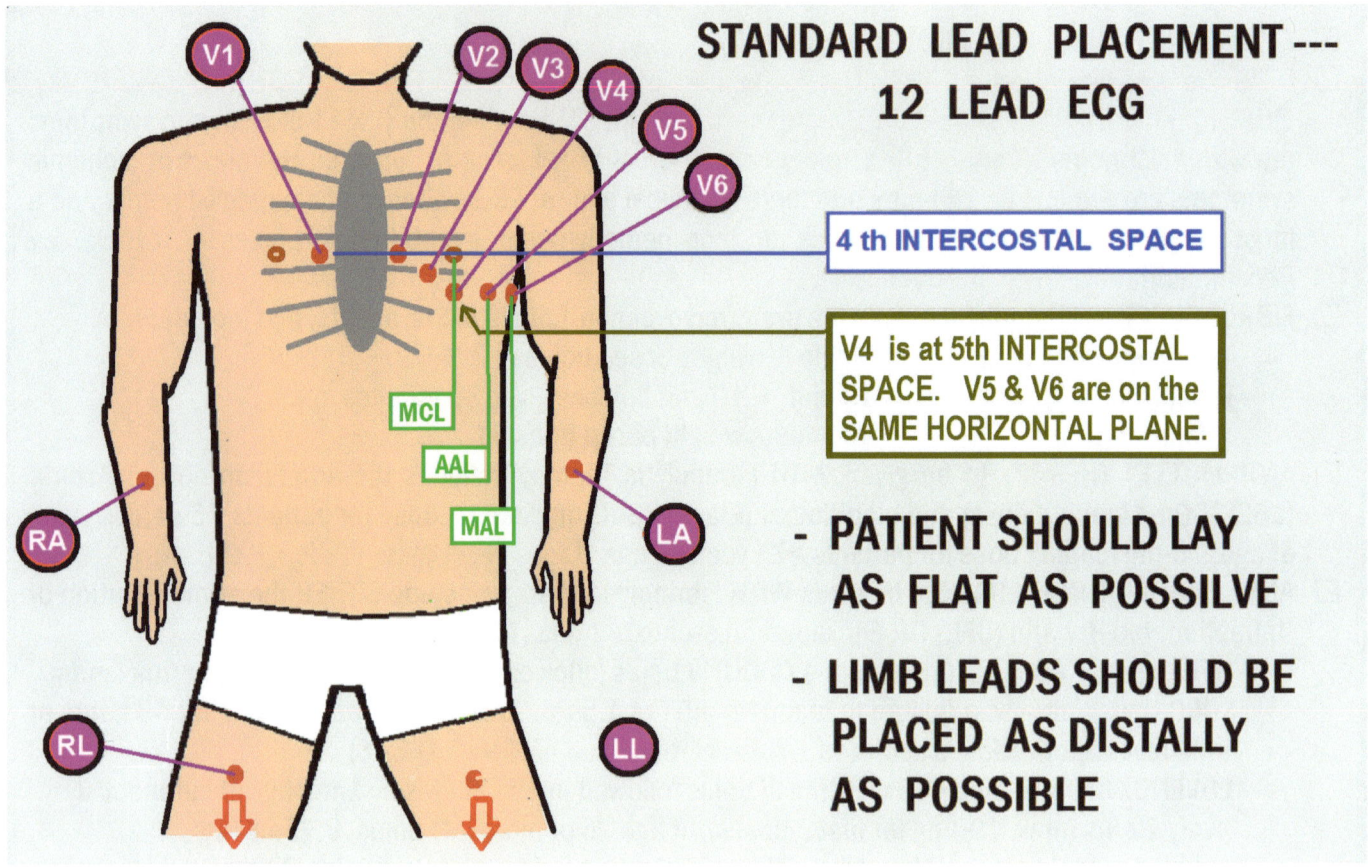

- ☐ Obtain and interpret 12 Lead ECG within 10 minutes of first patient contact (or chest pain onset).
- ☐ Limb leads should be on the limbs.
- ☐ When emergency circumstances dictate that limb leads be placed on patient's torso, the words "LIMB LEADS ON PATIENT'S TORSO" must be noted on the ECG.

EXPLANATION:

Recent AHA/ACC/HRS literature indicates QRS AMPLITUDE, Q WAVE DURATION, AXIS and WAVEFORM DEFLECTION can be altered when limb leads are placed on the patient's torso (Mason-Likar lead placement). Therefore every effort should be made to place limb leads on the limbs.

Proper lead placement of precordial Leads V1 and V2 are 4th intercostal space on opposite sides of the sternum. A common error is the superior misplacement of precordial Leads V1 and V2 in the second or third intercostal space. Incorrect placement of Leads V1 and V2 will result in: reduction of R wave amplitude (resulting in poor R wave progression) leading to misdiagnosis of previous anterior wall infarction, qR complexes in V1 and V2 resulting in misdiagnosis of previous septal wall infarction, or rSr complexes with T wave inversion, leading to misdiagnosis of obstructive pulmonary disease.

RIGHT SIDED ECG:

- ☐ OBTAIN A RIGHT-SIDED ECG IN ALL INSTANCES OF INFERIOR WALL MI.
- ☐ ST Elevation > 0.5mv (0.5mm) in V4R-V6R is considered ABNORMAL.
- ☐ NITRATES and DIEURETICS ARE CONTRAINDICATED IN RIGHT VENTRICULAR MI.

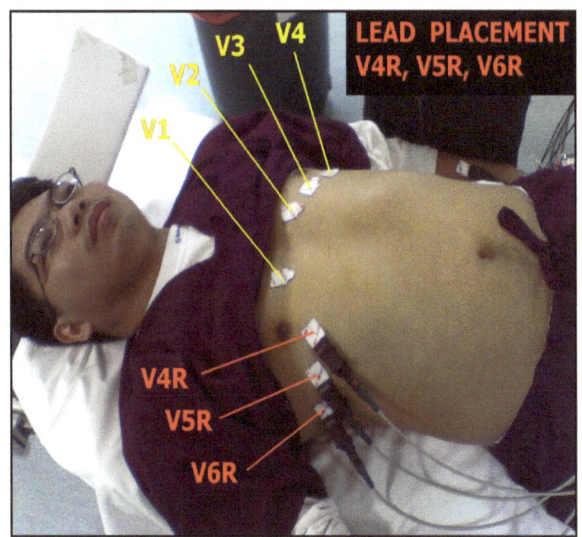

After the initial 12 Lead ECG is obtained, reposition the ECG electrodes for V1, V2 and V3 to the right precordium and place in the V4R, V5R and V6R positions, as illustrated in the photograph to the left. V4R should be located in the 5th intercostal space along the mid-clavicular line. V5R (and V6R) are located on the same horizontal plane as V4R. V5R is located along the Anterior Axillary Line, and V6R along the Mid-Axillary Line (mirror-opposite as their left-sided counterparts).

Right ventricular MI is commonly seen with Inferior MI, as the Right Coronary Artery provides blood supply to the inferior wall in 75-80% of the population.

POSTERIOR LEAD ECG:

- ☐ OBTAIN A POSTERIOR LEAD ECG on PATIENTS WITH ACS SYMPTOMS AND ST DEPRESSION IN ANTERIOR PRECORDIAL LEADS V1 - V4.
- ☐ ST ELEVATION > 0.5mv (0.5mm) in Leads V7 - V9 is considered ABNORMAL.

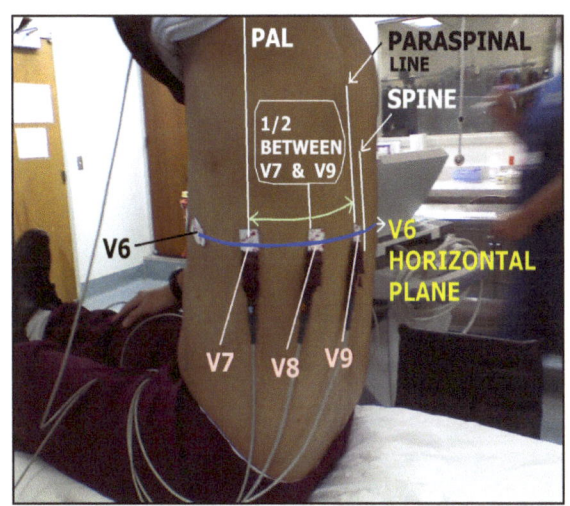

After the initial 12 Lead ECG is obtained, reposition the ECG lead wires for V4, V5 and V6 to the patient's back. As illustrated in the photograph to the left, all posterior leads will be placed on the same horizontal plane as Lead V6. V7 is placed along the posterior axillary line, V9 is placed just to the left of the spine, and V8 is centered between V7 and V9.

ST Depression in the anterior precordial leads (V1 - V4) could indicate anterior wall ischemia, anterior subendocardial MI (NSTEMI) or acute POSTERIOR WALL STEMI. To rule out POSTERIOR WALL STEMI, the Posterior Lead ECG should be obtained.

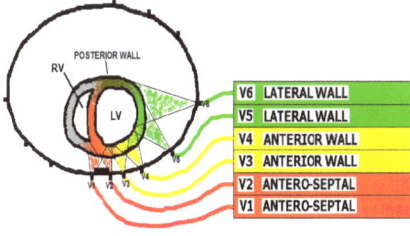

The standard 12 Lead ECG has two "blind spots" -- the RIGHT VENTRICLE and the POSTERIOR WALL. By obtaining both the Right-Sided and Posterior Lead ECG, more thorough evaluation is achieved.

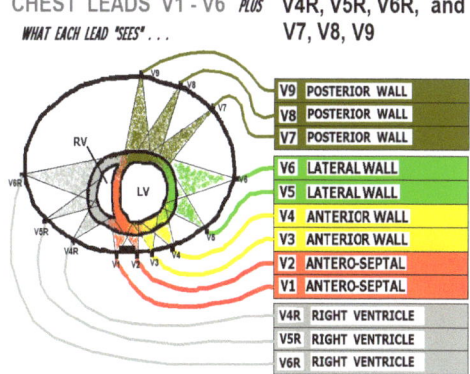

ECG EVALUATION for ACS -- FIRST: ASSESS WIDTH of QRS complexes

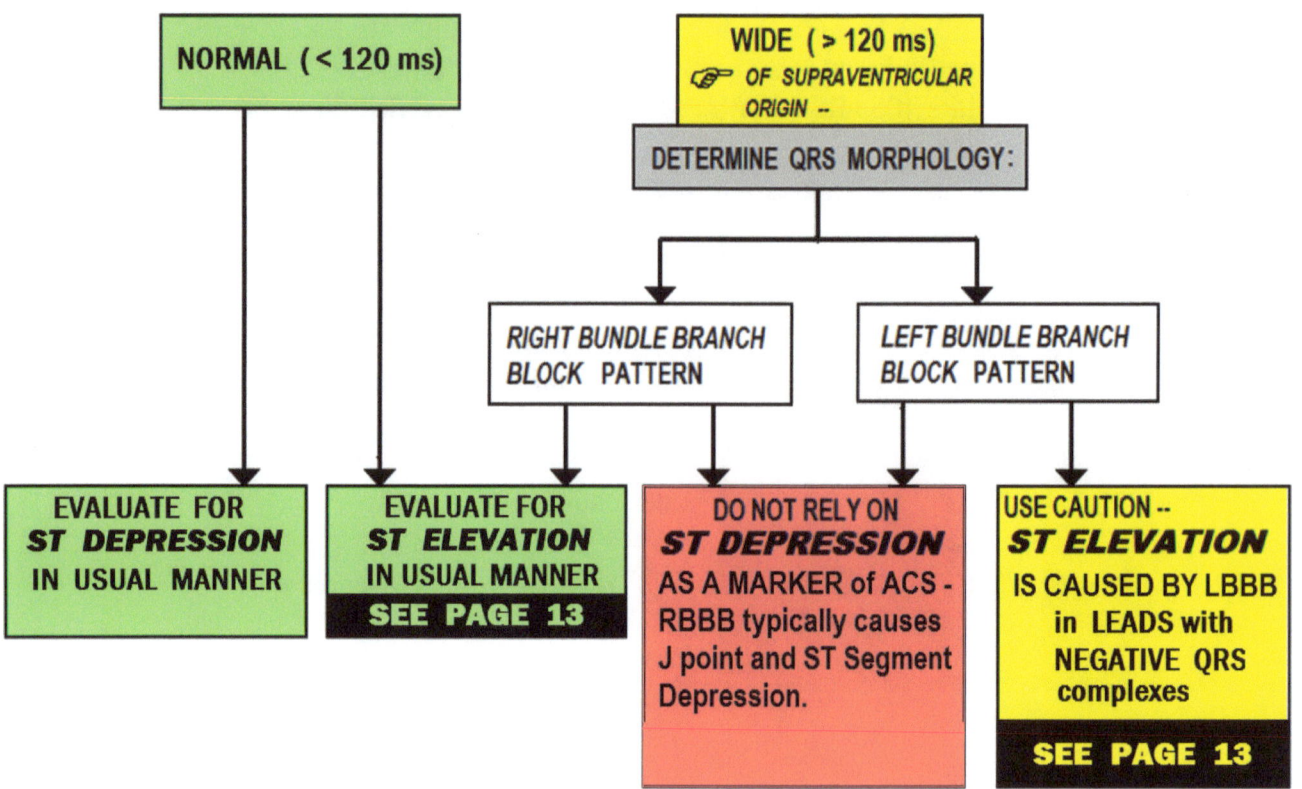

EXPLANATION:

Simply stated, *"if it DEPOLARIZES abnormally, it REPOLARIZES abnormally."*

Conditions that increase QRS duration (e.g. Bundle Branch Blocks, Paced Rhythms, WPW, Hypertrophy, etc) result in *secondary repolarization abnormalities* which in turn alter the J Point, ST Segment and T wave -- the ECG structures used to evaluate for the presence of ACS.

Therefore the first consideration when evaluating the ECG for the presence of ACS is to note if QRS complexes are abnormally wide (>120ms). If QRS width is normal, proceed to evaluate J Points, ST Segments and T waves in the usual manner. If the QRS duration is 120ms or more, determine QRS morphology (RBBB vs LBBB) and follow specific recommendations outlined in the flowchart above.

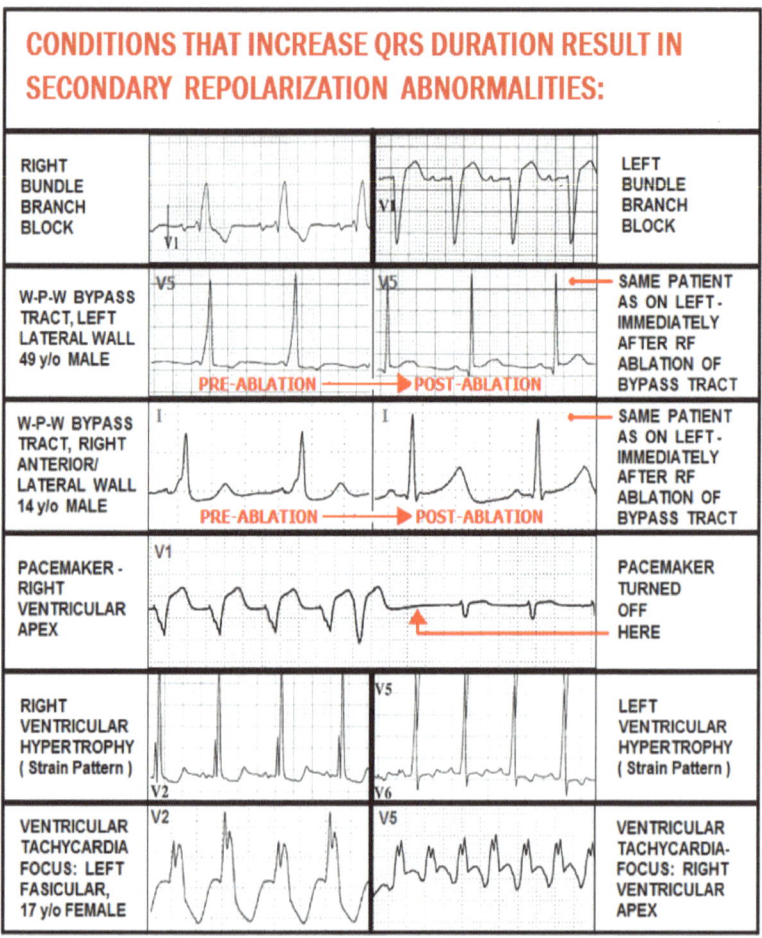

ECG EVALUATION for ACS: QRS WIDTH IS NORMAL (<120ms):

- ☐ **J POINT** GUIDELINES* for determination of ABNORMAL ST SEGMENT ELEVATION*:
    - V2, V3: males < 40 years old: 2.5mm
    - V2, V3: males age 40 and up: 2.0mm
    - V2, V3: all females: 1.5mm
    - Leads V3R - V6R: 0.5mm
    - Leads V7-V9: 0.5mm
    - ALL OTHER LEADS: 1.0mm

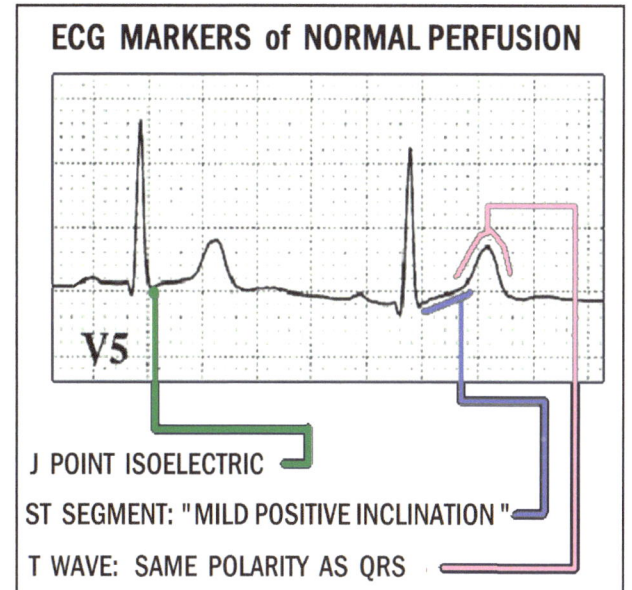

- ☐ **ST SEGMENT** should have "slight positive deflection," as seen in the image to the right.

- ☐ **T WAVES** normal criteria:
    - have rounded shape (NOT PEAKED)
    - generally have same polarity as QRS
    - not exceed amplitude of R wave
    - limb leads: not > 0.5mv (0.5mm)
    - precordial leads: not > 1.5mv (1.5mm)

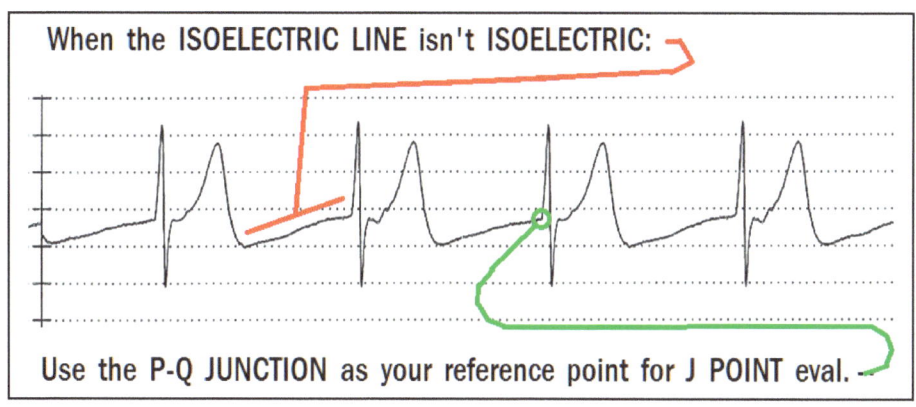

- ☐ If the TP segment (isoelectric line) is not flat, the P-Q Junction (point where PR segment and QRS coalesce) should be used as the reference point for evaluation of the J point for ST Segment deviation.

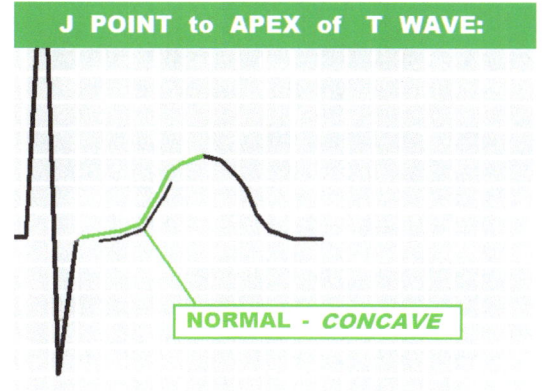

- ☐ Where the ST Segment and T wave merge, the shape should be CONCAVE, as indicated in the diagram to the right. When the waveform at this junction is FLAT or CONVEX, consider early-phase MI (see next page).

* Circulation 2009; Galen Wagner et al, AHA/ACCF/HRS Recommendations for the Standardization and Interpretation of the Electrocardiogram - Part VI: Acute Ischemia/Infarction

ECG EVALUATION for ACS: QRS WIDTH IS NORMAL (<120ms):

POSSIBLE INDICATORS of "EARLY PHASE" ACUTE MYOCARDIAL INFARCTION:

- **HYPERACUTE ("PEAKED") T WAVES:** Hyperacute T waves are associated with HYPERKALEMIA, TRANSMURAL ISCHEMIA, HYPERTROPHY and EARLY-PHASE ACUTE MI.
  - When HYPERACUTE T waves are noted globally, consider hyperkalemia
  - When HYPERACUTE T waves present in ONE TYPICAL ARTERIAL DISTRIBUTION (e.g.: Leads V1 - V4 = Left Anterior Descending Artery) consider TRANSMURAL ISCHEMIA or EARLY-PHASE ACUTE MI:

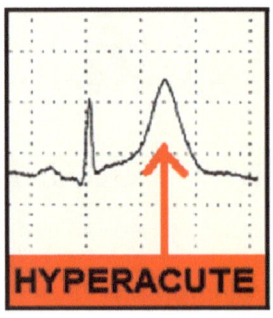 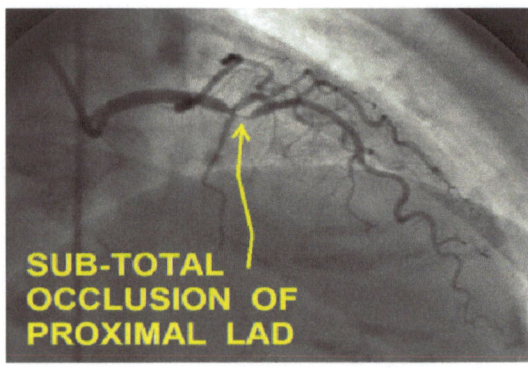 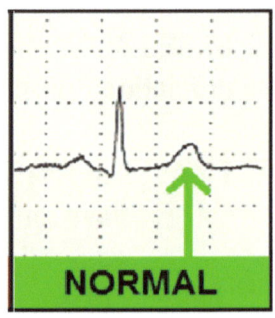

The ECG complex displayed to the left of this angiographic image illustrates that TRANSMURAL ISCHEMIA may result in the presence of HYPERACUTE T waves. Within minutes of the successful PCI of this sub-totally occluded PROXIMAL LAD lesion, the patient's T waves returned to NORMAL, as seen in the ECG complex to the above right.

- **FLAT and CONVEX JT-APEX SEGMENTS.** The atypical term "J-T Apex Segment" is used to identify the ST SEGMENT and approximately the first one half of the T wave.

  In the normal ECG with upright T waves, this segment is typically CONCAVE (as noted in the image at bottom of the previous page) and occasionally is noted to change to FLAT or CONVEX preceding STEMI, as seen in the examples to the right. These changes are also noted occasionally in the Cath Lab during PCI, when the balloon is inflated and temporarily obstructs coronary artery blood flow.

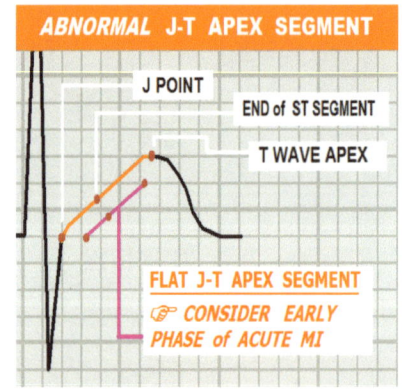
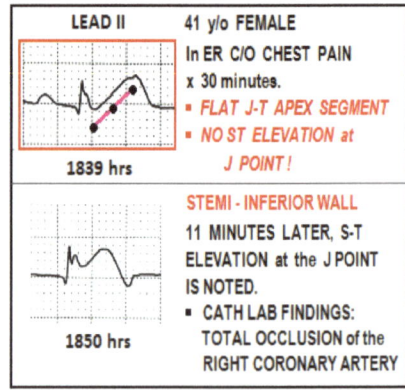
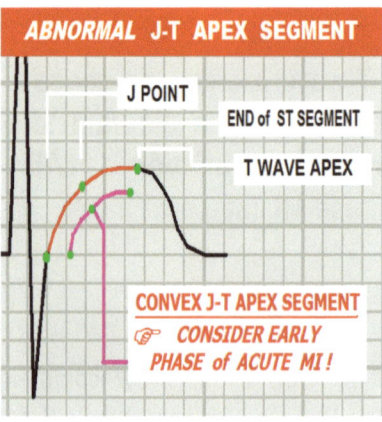
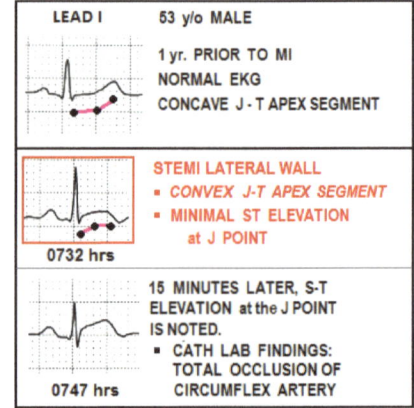

ST SEGMENT ELEVATION DURING STEMI:

Typical ST Elevation during STEMI can occur within seconds of total arterial occlusion, as noted in the example to the right, which was obtained during PCI in the Cardiac Cath Lab.

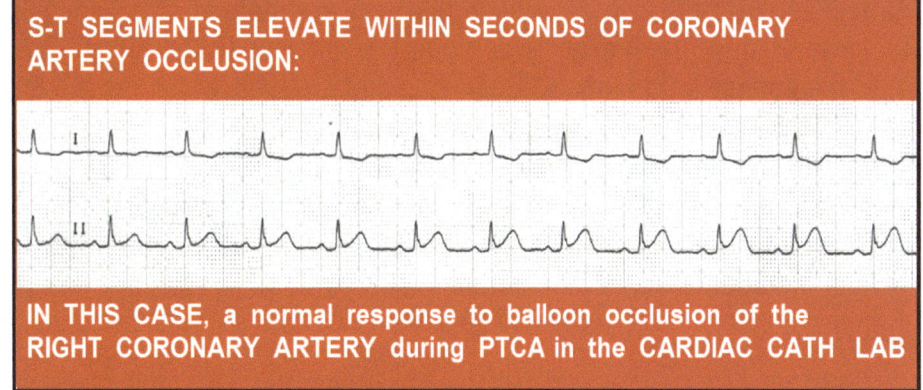

S-T SEGMENTS ELEVATE WITHIN SECONDS OF CORONARY ARTERY OCCLUSION:

IN THIS CASE, a normal response to balloon occlusion of the **RIGHT CORONARY ARTERY** during PTCA in the **CARDIAC CATH LAB**

During STEMI, the ST Segment elevates at the J Point. The amount of ST Elevation needed to meet STEMI criteria varies based on the ECG Lead (see "J Point Guidelines," top of PAGE 9). To be considered "POSITIVE for STEMI," traditional criteria states that there must be "ABNORMAL ST ELEVATION in TWO OR MORE CONTIGUOUS LEADS." However in the Cath Lab it is occasionally noted that patients with acute total coronary artery occlusion will present with *significant ST Elevation in ONE lead*, or *significant ST Elevation in two or more leads that were NOT contiguous* (e.g.: ST elevation in lead AVF and V3).

After the J Point, the ST Segment in true STEMI can be UPSLOPING, FLAT, or DOWNSLOPING, as noted in the samples below which were obtained from patients treated for STEMI in the Cath Lab:

PATTERNS of ST SEGMENT ELEVATION noted during STEMI

The following samples are from patients with ACUTE MI, as confirmed by discovery of total arterial occlusion in the Cardiac Cath Lab:

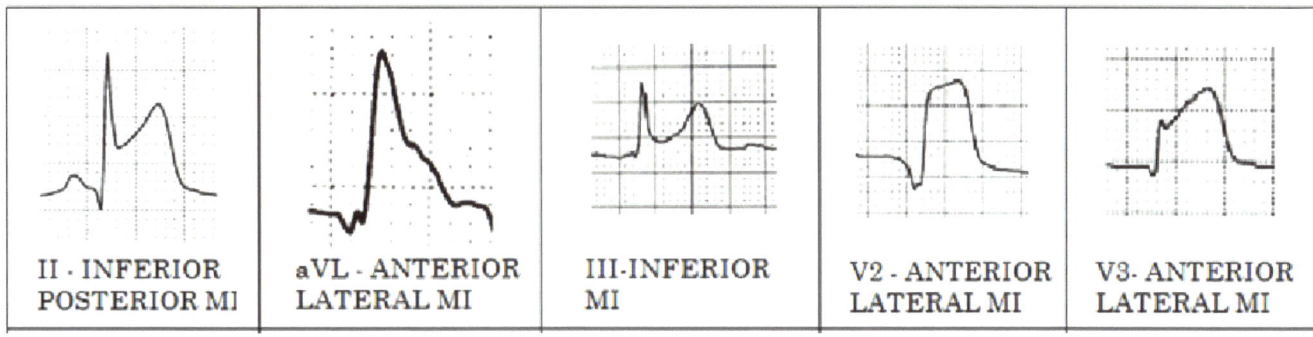

| II - INFERIOR POSTERIOR MI | aVL - ANTERIOR LATERAL MI | III - INFERIOR MI | V2 - ANTERIOR LATERAL MI | V3 - ANTERIOR LATERAL MI |

RECIPROCAL ST DEPRESSION in STEMI: The absence of ST Depression should not be used to rule out STEMI. Many STEMI patients do not have reciprocal ST Depression on their ECGs; the Anterior STEMI patient featured on page 24 does not. During ANTERIOR STEMI, when reciprocal ST depression is noted in Inferior Leads II, III and AVF, it's a reliable indicator that the proximal aspect of the Left Anterior Descending (LAD) artery is occluded; the zone of ischemia/infarction is larger than that of a mid-LAD occlusion. In cases of INFERIOR STEMI, when reciprocal ST depression is noted in Anterior Leads V1, V2 and sometimes V3, V4, it's a reliable indicator that there is Posterior ischemia/infarction as well. A general summary is that when reciprocal ST depression is noted during STEMI, the occlusion is located more proximally, and the zone of infarction / ischemia is larger than if no ST depression were present.

Differentiation of LEFT vs RIGHT BUNDLE BRANCH BLOCK

As indicated on page 8, conditions that cause abnormal QRS widening (e.g.: Bundle Branc Block, Wolff-Parkinson-White, Ventricular Hypertrophy) result in SECONDARY REPOLARIZATION ABNORMALITIES which alter the patient's J Points, ST Segments and T Waves, which are the ECG markers used to evalute for ACS. To futher complicate this issue, the changes differ between wide QRS complexes with RIGHT Bundle Branch Block (RBBB) aberrancy and LEFT Bundle Branch Block (LBBB) aberrancy. THEREFORE when QRS complexes are noted to be TOO WIDE -- 120ms (3mm) or wider -- we must determine if the wide QRS complex is of LBBB or RBBB morphology, and then apply the appropriate rules during ECG evaluation. There are several methods used to differentiate RBBB vs LBBB. We have selected two for their simplicity. BOTH methods utilize the QRS pattern of Lead V1:

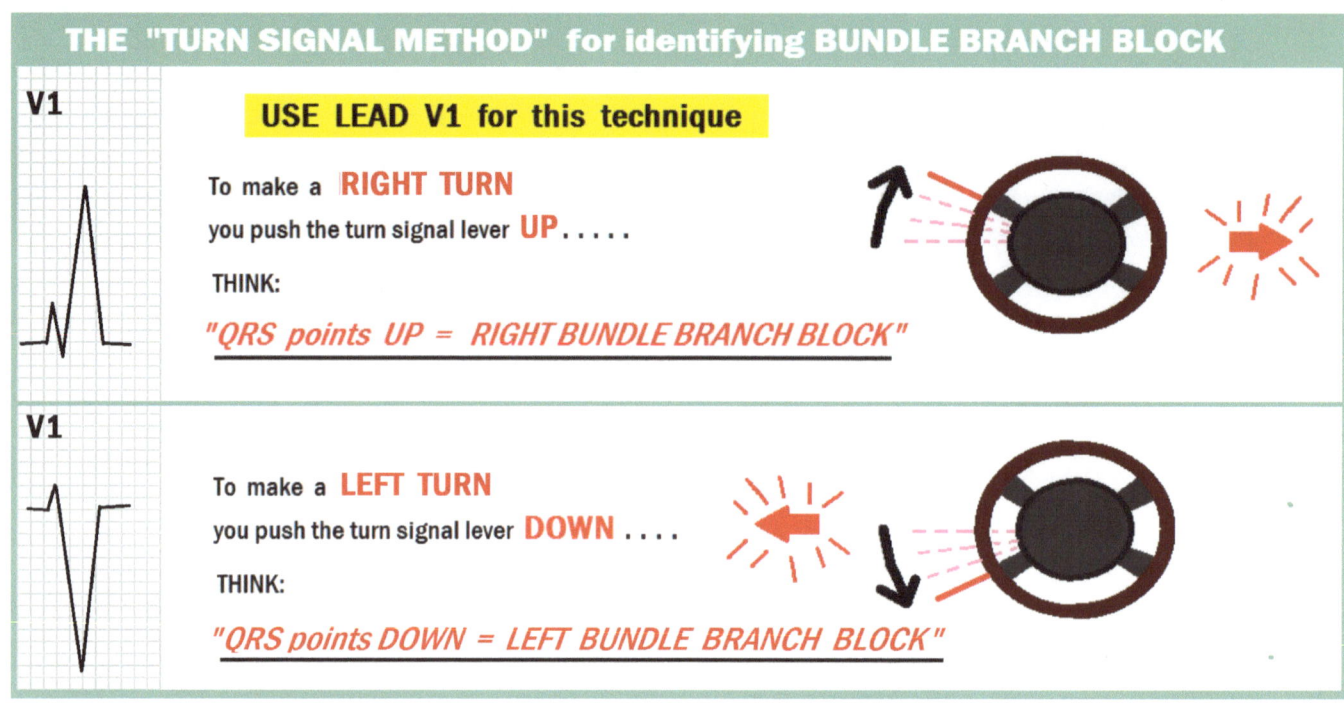

1. The Turn Signal Method. If the QRS complex is monophasic, we associate the rules of driving with ECG interpretation: every time you turn -- assuming that you're a courteous driver -- you use turn signals. When you wish to turn RIGHT, you push the turn signal lever UP and the RIGHT turn signal flashes. The analogous thought is that when the QRS is pointing UP, the QRS has RBBB morphology. When you wish to turn LEFT, you push the turn signal lever DOWN, and the left turn signal flashes -- so we associate a QRS that points down with LBBB. 's QRS in V1 is MAINLY NEGATIVE, the patient has a LBBB morphology.

2. Terminal Phase of QRS in Lead V1. The last method is also easy, and is what you should use when your patient's QRS is BiPhasic (has an equally positive and negative deflection), and the Turn Signal method won't work. With this method, simply look at the last deflection of the QRS complex and note if it is negative or positive. If it's negative, that favors LEFT bundle branch block; if it's positive, RIGHT Bundle Branch Block.

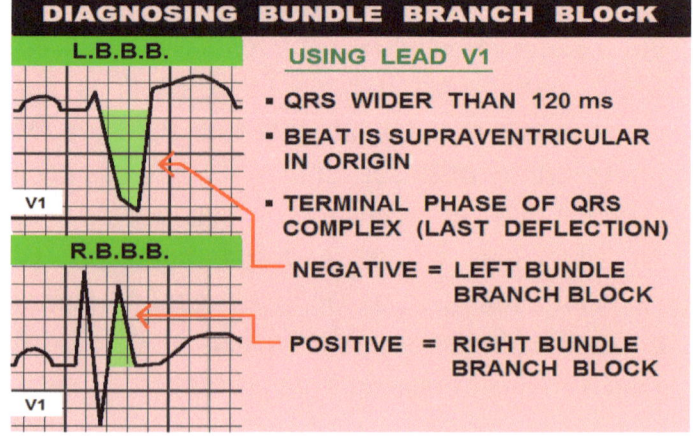

Identification of STEMI with the presence of BUNDLE BRANCH BLOCK:

RIGHT BUNDLE BRANCH BLOCK: Assess the ECG for ST Elevation in the usual manner -- transmural myocardial infarction in all regions of the myocardium will produce typical ST elevation despite the presence of RBBB. HOWEVER reciprocal ST Depression will be difficult to evaluate, as RBBB causes ST Depression and inverted T waves in the anterior precordial leads.

LEFT BUNDLE BRANCH BLOCK: causes more pronounced secondary ST and T wave changes, making diagnosis of STEMI challenging. The criteria listed below are from Circulation 2009; AHA/ACCF/HRS Recommendations for ECG interpretation in Acute Ischemia / Infarction, and Zimetbaum et al, NEJM 2003. The following ECG presentations noted in the presence of LBBB are consistent with Acute Myocardial Infarction:

- ☐ ST Elevation of 0.1mv (1mm) or more in Leads with POSITIVE QRS COMPLEXES.
- ☐ ST Elevation of 0.5mv (5mm) or more in Leads with NEGATIVE QRS COMPLEXES.
- ☐ ST Segment changes as compared with those of older ECGs with LBBB.
- ☐ Convex ST Segments

Note: New or presumably new LBBB should not be considered diagnostic of Acute Myocardial Infarction, as per 2013 ACCF/AHA Guidelines for Management of STEMI

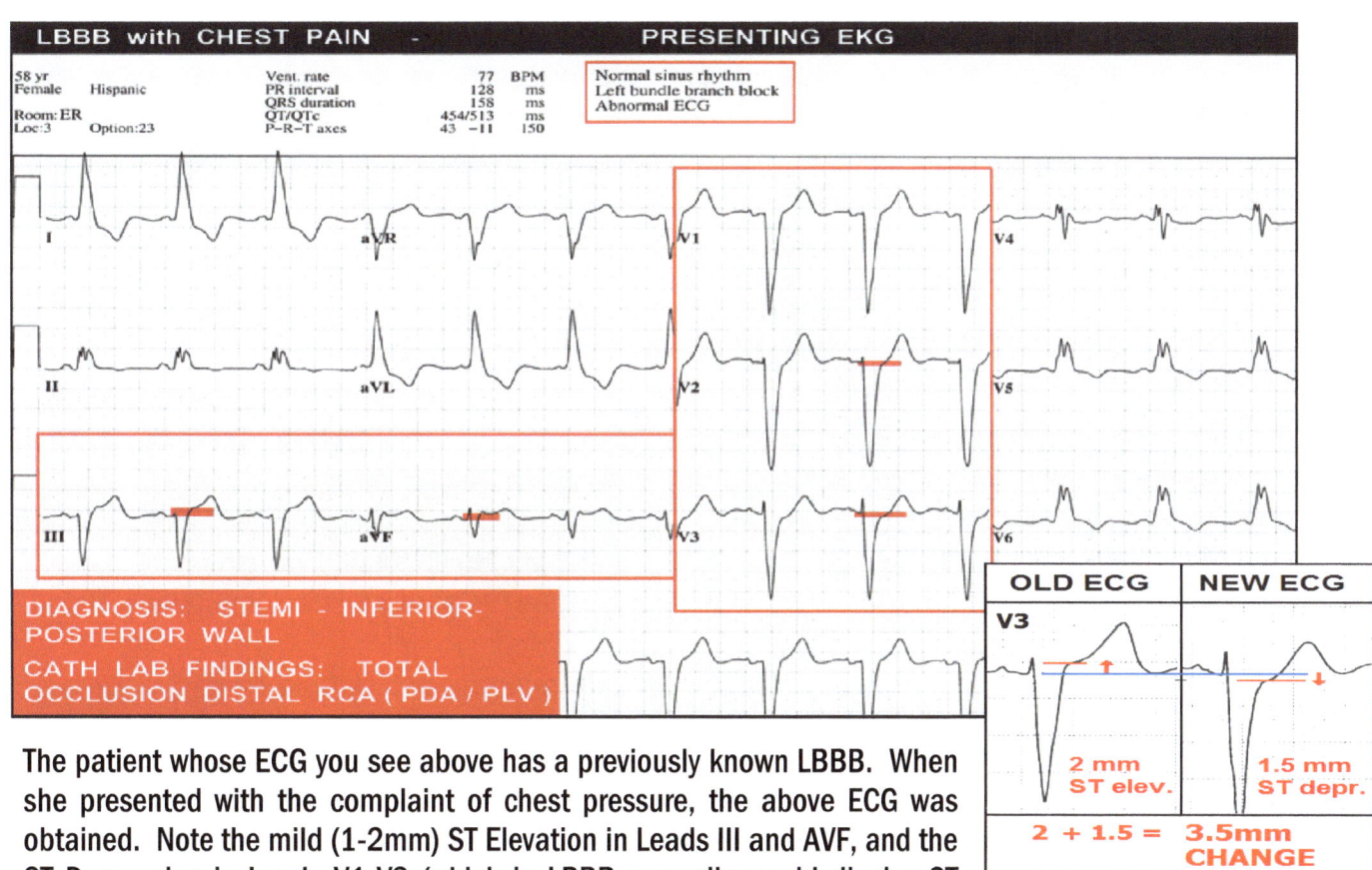

The patient whose ECG you see above has a previously known LBBB. When she presented with the complaint of chest pressure, the above ECG was obtained. Note the mild (1-2mm) ST Elevation in Leads III and AVF, and the ST Depression in Leads V1-V3 (which in LBBB normally would display ST Elevation). When compared to her ECG from a previous visit, the ST elevation in III and AVF are NEW, as is the ST Depression in V1-V3. This earned her a STAT visit to the Cath Lab, where we discovered a total thrombus occlusion of her distal RCA involving the PDA and PLV branches - which are consistent with Inferior ST Elevation and Posterior Wall MI. Also note the computer's misinterpretation of her ECG as "Normal."

REMOTE ISCHEMIC CONDITIONING:

Remote Ischemic Conditioning (RIC) is a procedure where brief and repeated cycles of non-lethal ischemia is introduced to targeted tissue (e.g.: a patient's extremity) which invokes a systemic protective cascade of cellular responses that reduce damage to mitochondria, reduce inflammatory responses to injury, and may significantly reduce damage during Acute MI and preserve LV function. Studies have been conducted where RIC is performed PRIOR to elective PCI (pre-conditioning), DURING PCI (per-conditioning), and AFTER PCI (post-conditioning).

It appears that in STEMI secondary to total coronary artery occlusion without collateralization, only modest preservation of LV function is described, with the protective effects being limited reducing damage associated with reperfusion immediately after PCI (post-conditioning).

However since many patients with STEMI are found to have significantly reduced (but not total occlusion) of blood flow PRIOR to PCI in the Cath Lab, (e.g.: patients with collateralization and/or partial thrombus) implementation of RIC to this group of patients may offer additional protective benefit. Since we often can't discern patients with TOTAL obstruction from those with PARTIAL obstruction, it is reasonable to administer RIC therapy to all STEMI patients when it won't delay PCI, such as during ambulance transport to the hospital or while in the ER awaiting arrival of the Cath Lab Team.

RIC appears to offer patients in the NSTEMI / Unstable Angina subset the most benefit prior to PCI, as there is often limited (TIMI Grade II) and adequate (TIMI Grade III) blood flow to the affected myocardial region. Therefore development of protocols that include utilization of RIC in this group of patients is a reasonable consideration.

RIC is not new: academic papers as far back as 1993 describe its use and benefits. Heusch et al (JACC 2015) suggests the following potential uses of RIC Preconditioning: Prior to elective PCI, Coronary Artery Bypass Graft and other open heart surgery procedures, carotid endarterectomy, aneurysm repair and other vascular surgeries; during episodes of unstable angina; protection of the brain and kidneys during episodes of ischemia. Other literature cites RIC benefits to the liver, intestines, lungs and pancreas.

Suggested PROTOCOL for REMOTE ISCHEMIC CONDITIONING (RIC):

1. STEMI patient - DON'T delay transport to hospital or cath lab to perform RIC.
2. Select upper extremity without previous vascular damage as you would for obtaining Blood Pressure (no history of mastectomy, shunts or other injury)
3. If unable to use upper extremity, a lower extremity may be used, with the same considerations listed above in item 1.
4. Apply Blood pressure cuff and inflate to 200mm/hg
5. Leave inflated for 5 minutes
6. Deflate - allow extremity to perfuse for 5 minutes
7. Repeat steps 3, 4 and 5 so that a TOTAL of FOUR CYCLES of five minutes of inflation and five minutes of deflation have been administered.

ACS RISK STRATIFICATION:

In cases of OBVIOUS STEMI, when your patient arrives clutching his chest, has pale diaphoretic skin and his ECG displays tombstone-shaped ST elevation, completion of an ACS Risk Stratification Score will most likely be of little value to your patient and will only delay reperfusion.

However in the NSTEMI ACS subgroup, utilization of an ACS Risk Stratification tool is considered a CLASS I Recommendation in the 2014 AHA/ACC Guidelines for Management of Patients with NSTEMI ACS.

Although specific delineation of additional diagnostic and therapeutic interventions for the NSTEMI/ UA patient is beyond the scope of this publication, we present the CLASS I Recommendations listed in the 2014 AHA/ACC NSTEMI ACS Guidelines to address the overlap often observed between the STEMI and NSTEMI/UA patient, and define the role of ACS Risk Stratification specific to these patient subsets.

2014 AHA/ACC NSTE-ACS Recommendations for patients without ST Elevation who exhibit symptoms highly suspicious for ACS include:

1. Obtain and interpret a 12 Lead ECG within 10 minutes of the patient's arrival (or onset of symptoms)
2. If the initial ECG is not diagnostic but the patient remains symptomatic and there is a high clinical suspicion of ACS, OBTAIN SERIAL ECGS at 15 - 30 MINUTE INTERVALS for the first hour and then repeated frequently and as the patient's symptoms change. ECG Monitoring with CONTINUOUS ST SEGMENT MONITORING, if available, is recommended in the lead(s) with abnormality noted on the 12 Lead ECG or leads that view each major coronary arterial distribution.
3. A STAT initial Troponin level followed by SERIAL Troponin Levels at 3 and 6 hours should be obtained. At these intervals it is also advisable to re-evaluate patient symptoms, obtain repeat 12 Lead ECGs and re-calculate ACS risk stratification scores.
4. Additional Troponin levels are indicated beyond 6 hours when Troponin levels are normal and changes on the ECG and/or the patient's symptoms confer a high index of suspicion for ACS.
5. Risk Scores should be used to assess prognosis in patients with NSTEMI / ACS and low risk chest pain, and are useful in the management of the patient.

With respect to selection of an appropriate ACS Risk Stratification model, we recommend the HEART Score due to multiple recent evidence based studies that demonstrate HEART's superior sensitivity, specificity and overall accuracy in predicting the presence of obstructive coronary artery disease in both the high and low risk populations.

In a prospective validation study consisting of 2,440 randomly selected patients (International Journal of Cardiology 2013) the HEART Score was compared to the TIMI and GRACE scores for its capability to accurately predict the occurrence of Major Adverse Cardiac Events (MACE) within 6 weeks. MACE included Acute MI, the need for PCI or CABG or death due to any cause.

The HEART Score achieved a C-statistic of 0.83, the TIMI 0.75, and GRACE achieved a c-statistic of 0.70. (The C-statistic is a measure of the discriminatory power of a predictive model. A score of "1.00" would mean it is PERFECT -- and a 0.50 is the same as a "50-50 coin toss").

The graph to the right demonstrates the superior predictive power of the HEART Score in the low risk patient population as well as the in the high risk population.

Predictive Values of LOW Scores:

In patients with LOW HEART scores (0-3) there was only a 1.7% incidence of MACE as compared to low TIMI scores (0-1) with a 2.8% incidence of MACE, and GRACE low scores, 2.9%

Predictive Values of HIGH Scores:

Only HEART and TIMI scores demonstrated a significant correlation between high scores and MACE, with HEART once again taking 1st place: Patients with HEART Scores of 7-10, the incidence of MACE was 50.0%, and with high TIMI Scores (6-7) the MACE Incidence was 42.5%

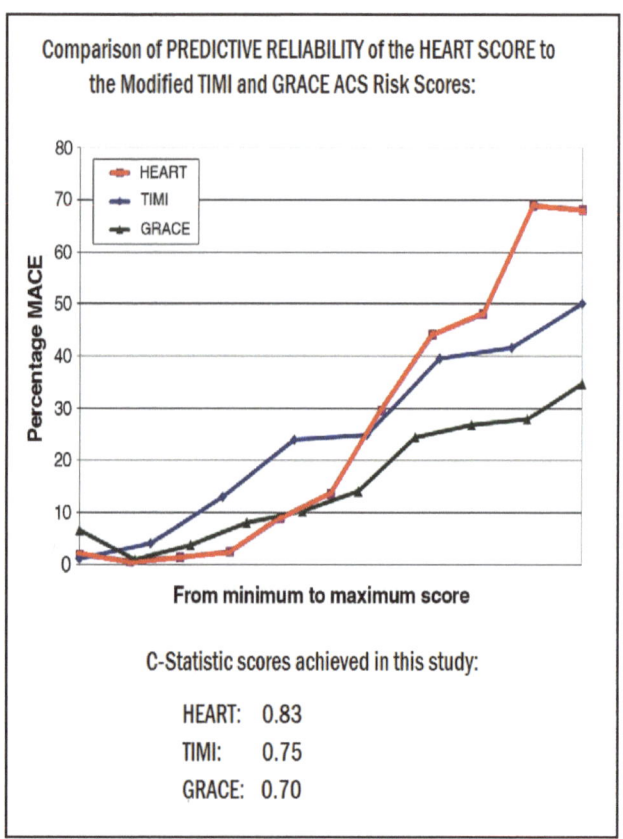

Comparison of PREDICTIVE RELIABILITY of the HEART SCORE to the Modified TIMI and GRACE ACS Risk Scores:

C-Statistic scores achieved in this study:

HEART: 0.83
TIMI: 0.75
GRACE: 0.70

HEART

HEART score for chest pain patients

History	Highly suspicious	2
	Moderately suspicious	1
	Slightly suspicious	0
ECG	Significant ST-deviation	2
	Non specific repolarisation disturbance / LBTB / PM	1
	Normal	0
Age	≥ 65 years	2
	> 45 and < 65 years	1
	≤ 45 years	0
Risk factors	≥ 3 risk factors or history of atherosclerotic disease*	2
	1 or 2 risk factors	1
	No risk factors known	0
Troponin	≥ 3x normal limit	2
	> 1 and < 3x normal limit	1
	≤ 1x normal limit	0
		Total

*Risk factors for atherosclerotic disease:

Hypercholesterolemia Cigarette smoking
Hypertension Positive family history
Diabetes Mellitus Obesity

The overall summary of the HEART Score is that is demonstrates superior predictive power over the TIMI Score in both ends of the scale. Patients with high HEART Scores had higher incidence of needing PCI or CABG, and those with lower HEART Scores had much lower rates of MACE.

According to Circulation Outcomes 2015, Mahler et al describe a new Low Risk Chest Pain strategy that utilizes the HEART Score combined with two Troponin measurements (0 and 3 hours). The strategy, referred to as The HEART Pathway, demonstrated that patients in the HEART Pathway Group of the study had a shorter Length of Stay in the hospital than those in the Usual Care group, *and NONE of the patients in the HEART Pathway Group suffered MACE at 30 days in contrast to 19 in the Usual Care Group who did.*

Correlation of ECG Leads with Coronary Anatomy

FIRST, INTERPRET THE ECG, THEN...
- IDENTIFY THE AREA OF THE HEART AFFECTED BY THE MI
- RECALL THE ARTERY WHICH SERVES THAT REGION...
- RECALL OTHER STRUCTURES SERVED BY THAT ARTERY...
- ANTICIPATE FAILURE OF THOSE STRUCTURES...
- **INTERVENE APPROPRIATELY!**

The ability to correlate ST segment abnormalities on a patient's ECG with common coronary artery anatomy is vital to understanding the physiological changes that occur during Acute MI. This knowledge facilitates a practitioner's ability to accurately anticipate specific complications *and prepare for intervention* BEFORE they occur.

Two coronary arterial configurations account for approximately 90 percent of the population, and in this book are referred to as *common coronary arterial anatomy*. Right Coronary Artery (RCA) dominant systems are found in 75-80% of the population, and Left Circumflex (Cx) dominant systems in 10-15%. The term "dominant" translates *to "the artery that supplies blood to the inferior wall of the left ventricle and the AV node."* These differences are illustrated in the images below:

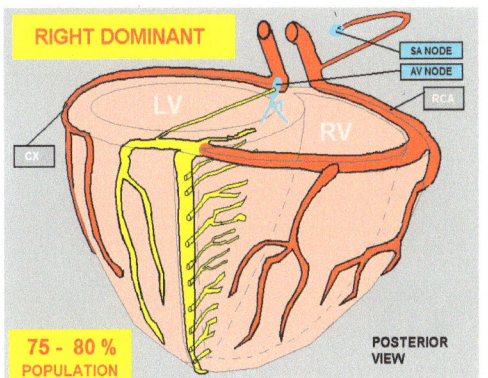
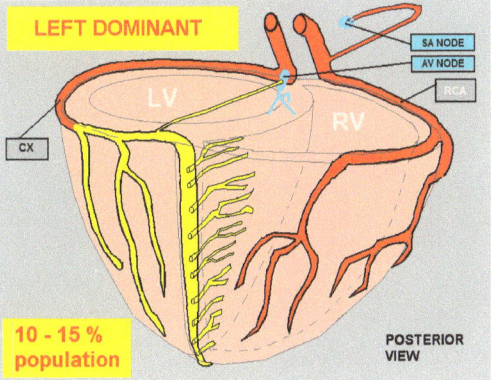

The table below pertains to patients with common coronary arterial anatomy. When these patients present with ST elevation in the leads listed, correlate these leads with the coronary artery that is most likely occluded and the associated structures that they perfuse: anticipate failure of these structures and be prepared to intervene appropriately. Detailed information about each type of MI and its management is featured in this book on pages 18 - 35.

	ECG Leads:	Associated Region:	Coronary Artery:	Structures at Risk:	Example(s) on Pages:
All Patients	V1 - V4	Anterior and Septal walls of LV	Left Anterior Descending (LAD) Atery	- 35 - 45% of LV muscle mass - Bundle of HIS - Bundle Branches	24 - 27
RCA Dominant	V5 - V6	Lateral wall LV, approx. 50% Posterior wall	Circumflex (Cx) (non - dominant)	- 20 - 30% LV muscle mass - Sinus Node (rare)	22 - 23
RCA Dominant	II, III, AVF	Inferior Wall, approx. 50% Posterior wall	Right Coronary Artery (RCA)	- SA Node - Right Ventricle - AV Node	28 - 31
Cx Dominant	V5 - V6 + II, III, AVF	Lateral wall of LV Posterior Wall (all) Inferior Wall	Circumflex (Dominant)	- 45-55% LV muscle mass - SA Node (rare) - AV Node	32 - 33

The remaining 10% of the population have one of several less common coronary arterial anatomic configurations, (e.g.: the anomalous "single" coronary artery). In cases of STEMI the ECG may demonstrate ST elevation in lead sets that are unusual, and complications can be difficult to predict. For more information see "<u>12 Lead ECG Intepretation in ACS with Case Studies from the Cardiac Cath Lab,</u>" listed on page 38.

- ☑ **ST ELEVATION ≥ 0.5mv (0.5mm) AVR**
- ☑ **ST ELEVATION or ST DEPRESSION in MOST or ALL LEADS**
- ☑ **ST ELEVATION in LEADS AVR, I, and AVL**
- ☑ **WIDENING of QRS COMPLEXES**
- ☑ **qR I, AVL + rS II, III + LEFT AXIS DEVIATION**
  (QRS -45 to -90 degrees)

ST SEGMENT ELEVATION
ST SEGMENT DEPRESSION

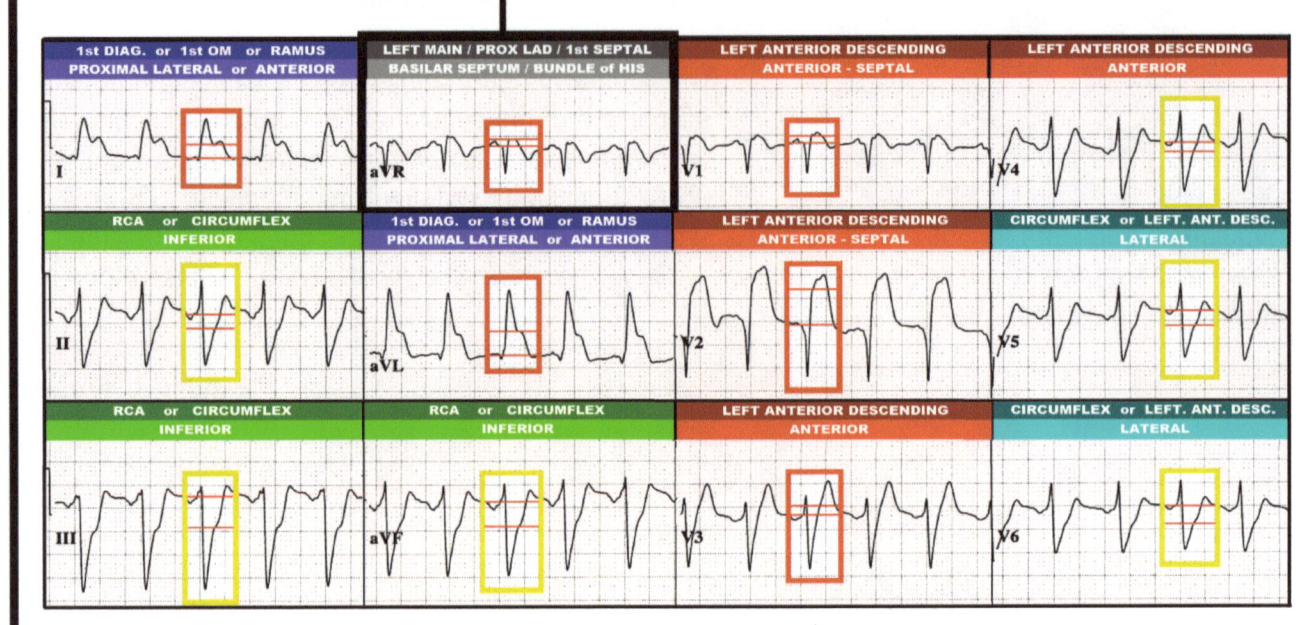

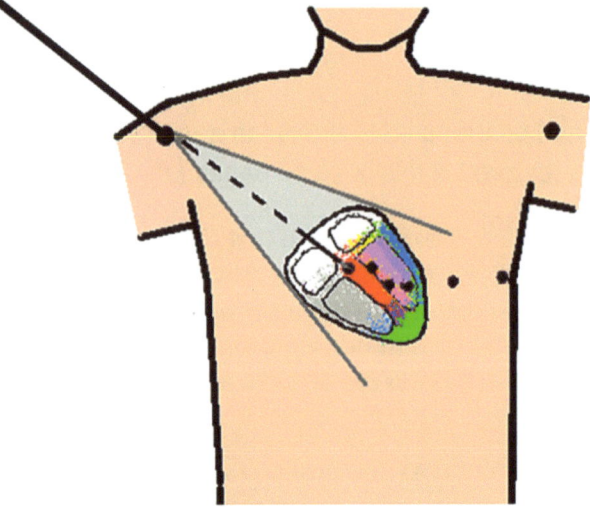

Lead AVR views the BASILAR SEPTUM, the region perfused by the FIRST SEPTAL PERFORATOR originating from the PROXIMAL LAD.

ST ELEVATION in Lead AVR during STEMI is associated with ARTERIAL OCCLUSION of the LEFT MAIN CORONARY ARTERY or the (very) PROXIMAL Left Anterior Descending Artery.

ST Elevation in Lead AVR greater than 0.5mm is an indicator that the obstruction is proximal to the 1st Septal Perforator arising from the proximal Left Anterior Descending Artery (LAD), as is ST Elevation in Leads I & AVL; these findings are commonly noted in GLOBAL MI secondary to obstruction of the LEFT MAIN CORONARY ARTERY. THE PRECORDIAL LEADS may exhibit ST Elevation, but it is common to see isoelectric ST segments or a combination of ST elevation and depression caused by the COMPETING FORCES of ANTERIOR vs. POSTERIOR WALL MI. Widening of QRS Complexes during STEMI is an ominous sign and indicates there is no-flow to the Bundle of His and proximal Bundle Branches. An Anterior Fascicular Block pattern is nearly always present: The QRS is POSITIVE (qR) in Leads I and AVL, and NEGATIVE (rS) in II, III and sometimes AVF. In the frontal plane, the QRS Axis is typically -45 to -90 (Left Axis Deviation). Typically every lead displays ST elevation or depression.

ECG presentation consistent with:

GLOBAL MI
secondary to obstruction of the LEFT MAIN CORONARY ARTERY (LMCA).

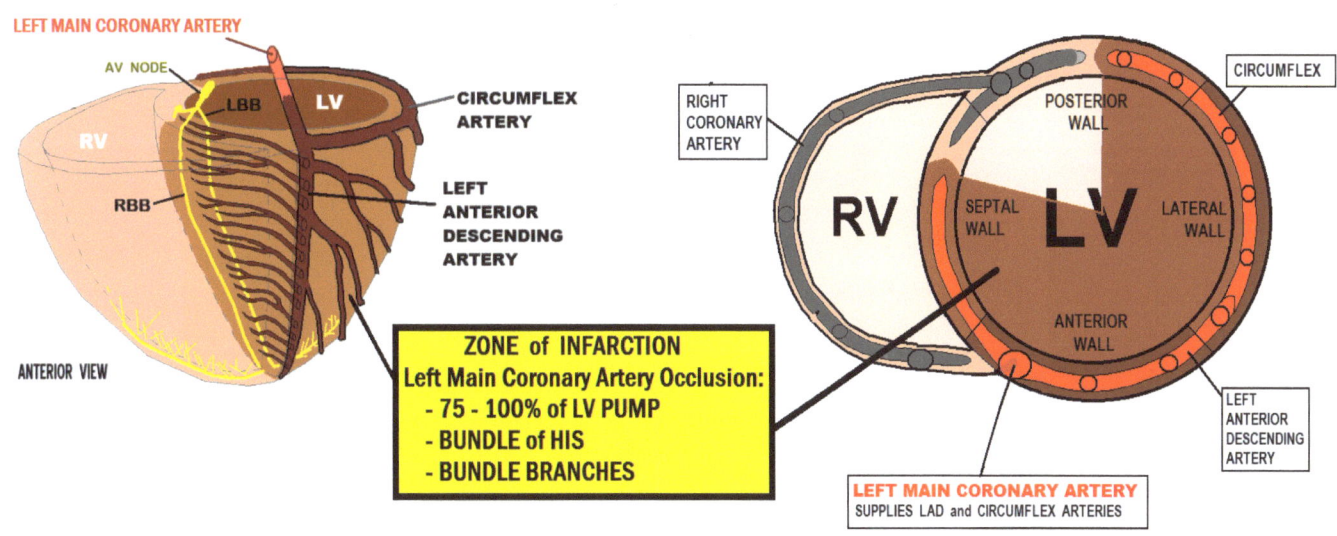

ANTICIPATED COMPLICATIONS of GLOBAL STEMI & POSSIBLE INDICATED INTERVENTIONS:	
- IMMINENT CARDIAC ARREST	BCLS / ACLS
- 75% MORTALITY RATE	PATIENT NEEDS IMMEDIATE REPERFUSION: the standard "90 minute Door-To-PCI time" is TOO LONG for this patient.
- PROFOUND PUMP FAILURE and CARDIOGENIC SHOCK	INOTROPE THERAPY: -DOPAMINE / LEVOPHED / DOBUTAMINE - INTRA-AORTIC BALLOON PUMP (use caution with fluid challenges due to PULMONARY EDEMA)
- CARDIAC DYSRHYTHMIAS (VT / VF)	ACLS (antiarrhythmics). ACLS therapy will most likely be INEFFECTIVE if IMMEDIATE REPERFUSION is not achieved.
- PULMONARY EDEMA	- CPAP - ET INTUBATION (use caution with diuretics due to pump failure and hypotension)

- ☑ **ST ELEVATION in LEAD AVR**
- ☑ **ST DEPRESSION in 8 OR MORE LEADS**
- ☑ **NOT CLASSIFIED as "STEMI" DUE TO ST ELEVATION PRESENT IN LEAD AVR ONLY TROPONIN MAY BE ELEVATED (NSTEMI) or NORMAL.**

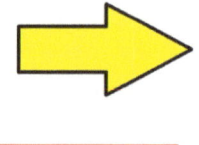

ST SEGMENT ELEVATION
ST SEGMENT DEPRESSION

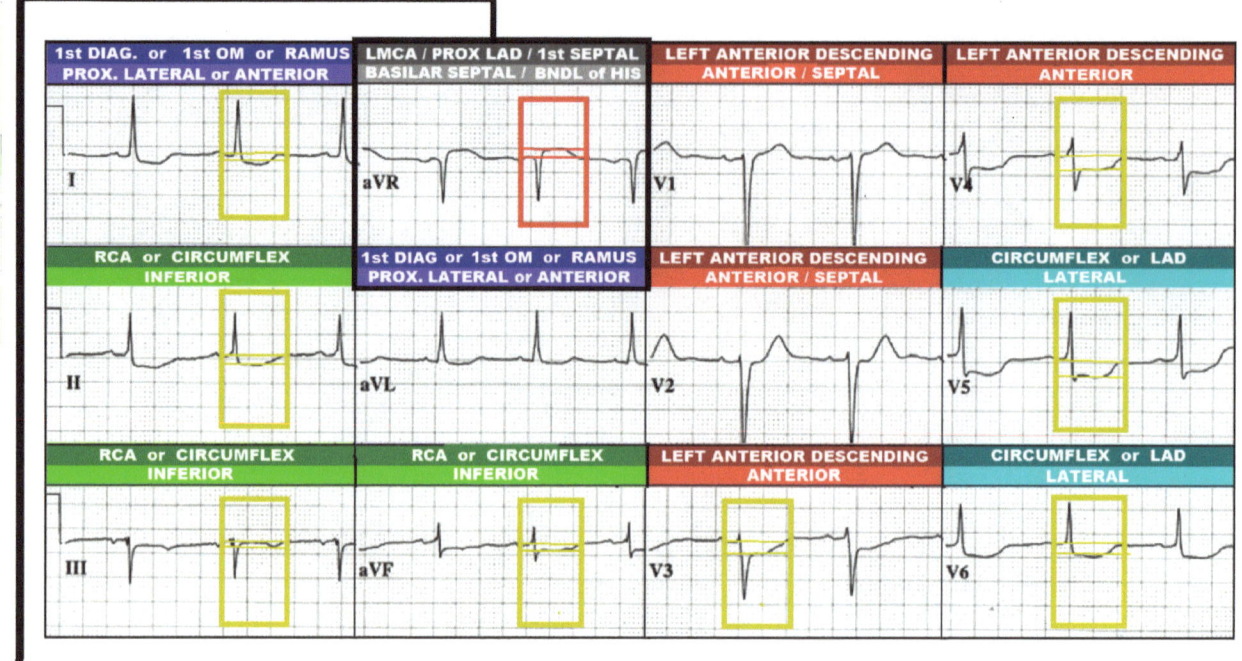

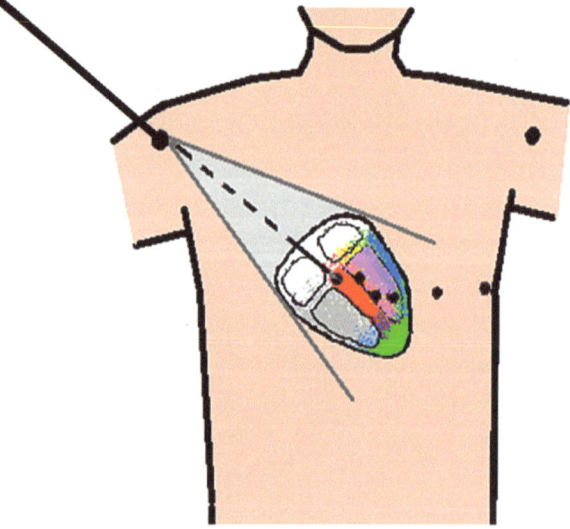

Lead AVR views the BASILAR SEPTUM, the region perfused by the FIRST SEPTAL PERFORATOR originating from the PROXIMAL LAD.

Patients with PRIMARY ST ELEVATION in Lead AVR and GLOBAL ISCHEMIA (ST - DEPRESSION in 8 or more ECG Leads) who experience ANGINA at REST have a 75% incidence of CRITICAL STENOSIS of the LEFT MAIN CORONARY ARTERY or SEVERE TRIPLE- VESSEL DISEASE *

* 1. Circulation 2009: AHA/ACCF/HRS Recommendations for the Standardization and Interpretation of the ECG: Part VI: Acute Ischemia / Infarction;
 2. Circulation 2013: ACCF/AHA Guidelines for Management of STEMI

ECG presentation consistent with:

GLOBAL ISCHEMIA

secondary to severe stenosis of the LEFT MAIN CORONARY ARTERY (LMCA) and/or ADVANCED TRIPLE-VESSEL DISEASE. Typically Coronary Artery Bypass Graft (CABG) surgery is indicated.

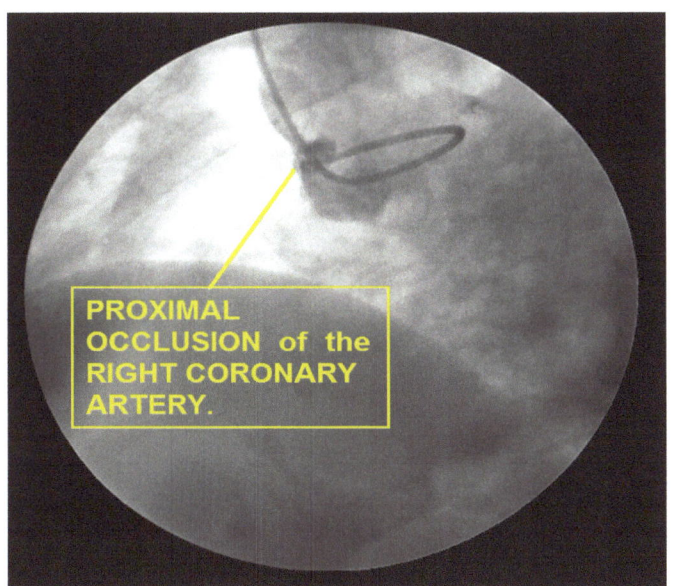 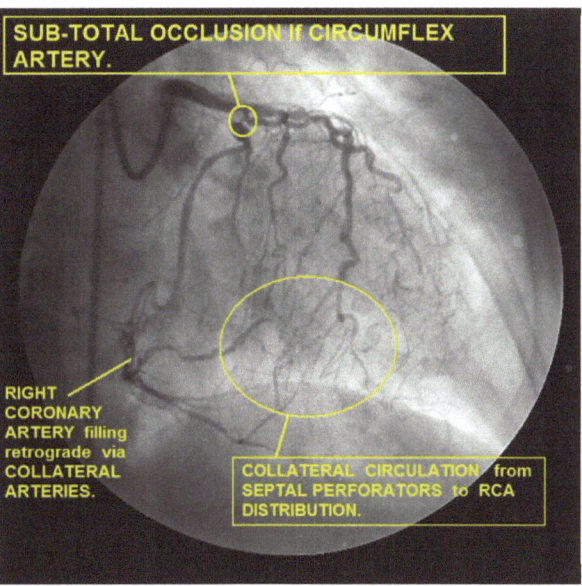

The angiographic images above are those of the patients whose 12 Lead ECG is featured on the opposite page. She underwent immediate 4 vessel coronary bypass surgery.

ANTICIPATED COMPLICATIONS of GLOBAL ISCHEMIA with POSSIBLE NSTEMI -- INTERVENTIONS to be CONSIDERED:	
Patients with CHEST PAIN at REST and this ECG presentation have a 75% incidence of severe LMCA STENOSIS and/or TRIPLE - VESSEL DISEASE -- in such cases Coronary Artery Bypass Surgery (CABG) is frequently indicated.	PREHOSPITAL: if patient has no hospital preference consider transport to Chest Pain Center WITH Open Heart Surgery capabilites IF nearby. HOSPITAL: consider use of SHORT-ACTING intravenous GP IIb/IIIa receptor agonists
- ACTIVE CHEST PAIN	ACUTE CHEST PAIN PROTOCOL
- ISCHEMIA - CONSIDER DYSRHYTHMIAS	ACLS PROTOCOL
- INCREASED PROBABILITY of IMMINENT MYOCARDIAL INFARCTION	1. AGGRESSIVE SERIAL TROPONIN and SERIAL ECG PROTOCOLS (2014 AHA /ACC / NSTE-ACS Guidelines) 2. Positive TROPONIN: consider STAT / early Cardiac Catheterization

☑ **PRIMARY ST ELEVATION in LEADS V5 & V6, may extend to LEADS I, AVL, V4, V3**

☑ **Possible ST Depression Leads II, III, & AVF**

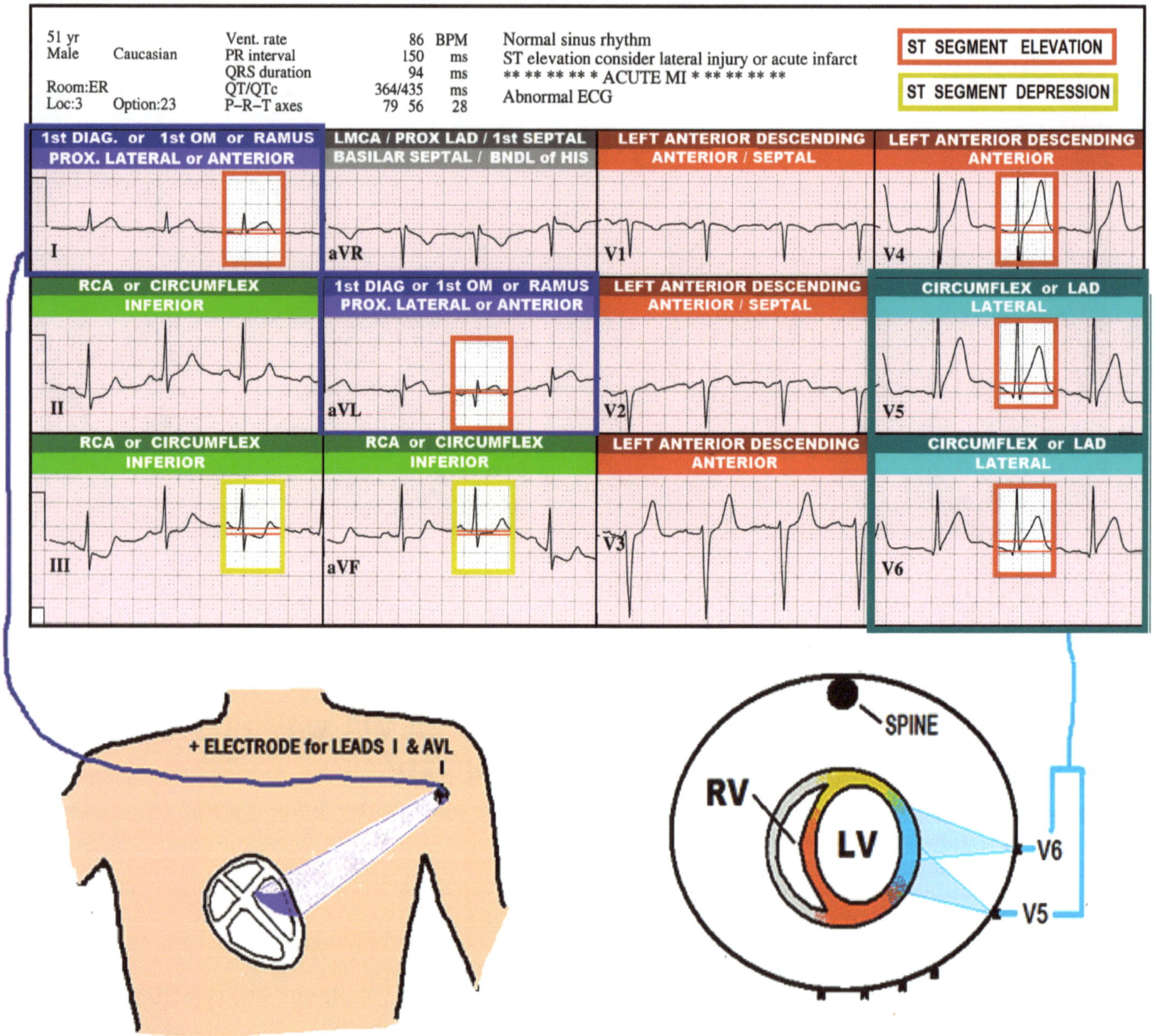

Leads I and AVL view the **ANTERIOR - LATERAL JUNCTION** of the LEFT VENTRICLE

Leads V5 and V6 view the **LATERAL WALL** of the LEFT VENTRICLE

ECG presentation consistent with:

LATERAL WALL MI

secondary to obstruction of a NON-DOMINATNT CIRCUMFLEX Artery (Cx).

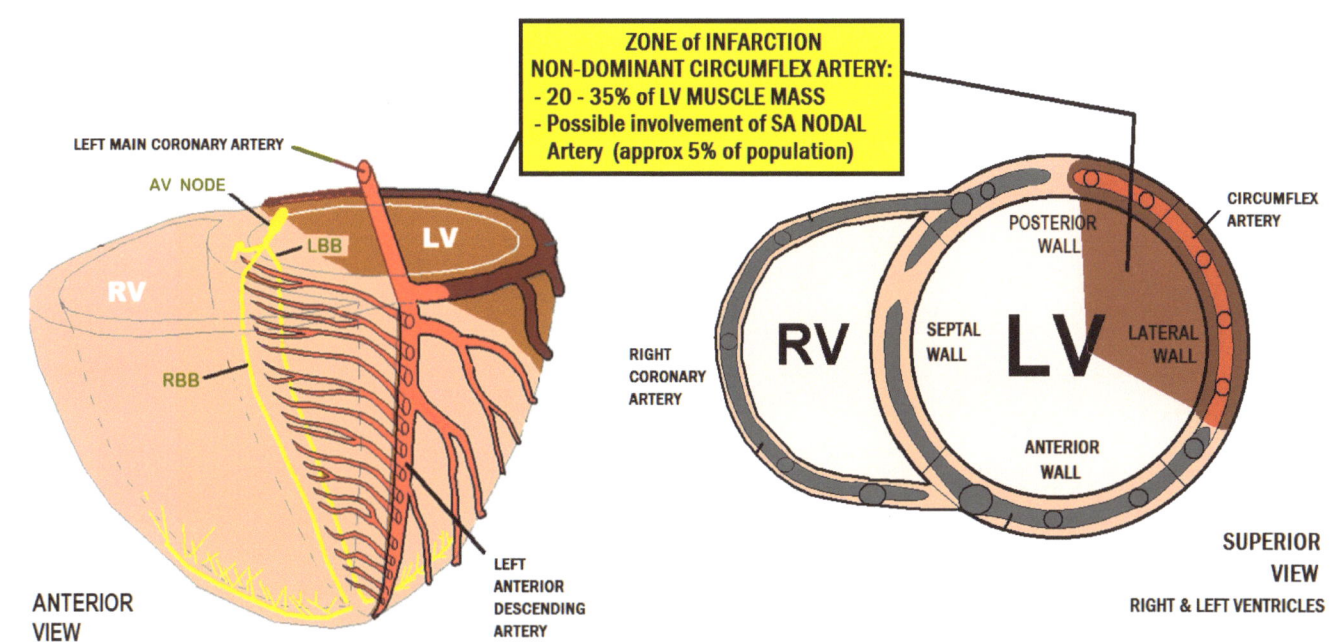

ANTICIPATED COMPLICATIONS of LATERAL WALL STEMI & POSSIBLE INDICATED INTERVENTIONS:	
- CARDIAC ARREST	BCLS / ACLS
- CARDIAC DYSRHYTHMIAS (VT / VF)	ACLS
- MILD / MODEREATE PUMP FAILURE / HYPOTENSION:	INOTROPE THERAPY: -DOPAMINE / LEVOPHED / DOBUTAMINE LOW VOLUME FLUID CHALLENGE (use caution with fluid challenges - ASSESS LUNG SOUNDS prior to any fluid challenge to rule out presence of PULMONARY EDEMA)
- SA NODAL FAILURE (approx 5 % of population - SA nodal artery originates from Left Circumflex Artery).	ATROPINE

Scroll through pages in this section to find the 12 Lead ECG with ST PATTERNS which most closely resemble that of your patient's ECG

☑ **ST ELEVATION in Leads V1 - V4, may extend into V5, V6**

☑ **No Reciprocal ST DEPRESSION in Leads II, III or AVF**

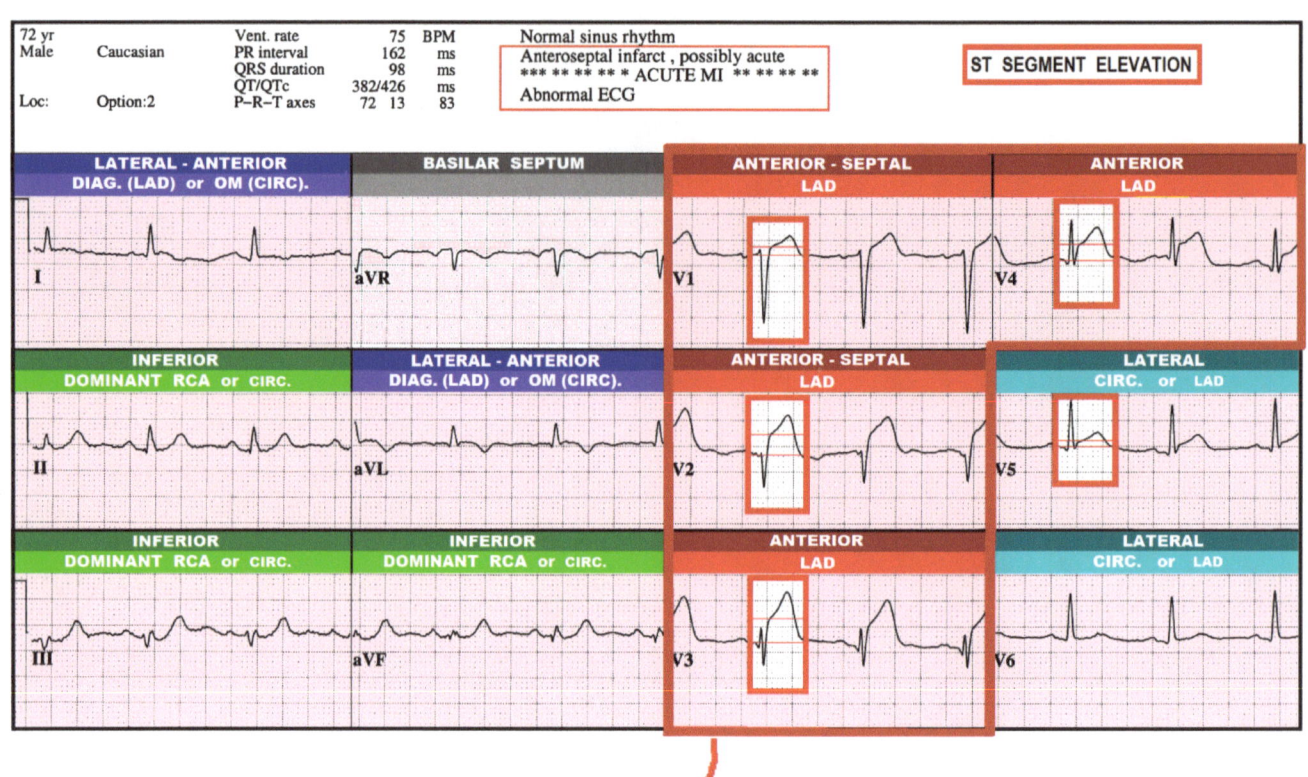

V1 - V4 VIEW the ANTERIOR - SEPTAL WALL of the LEFT VENTRICLE.

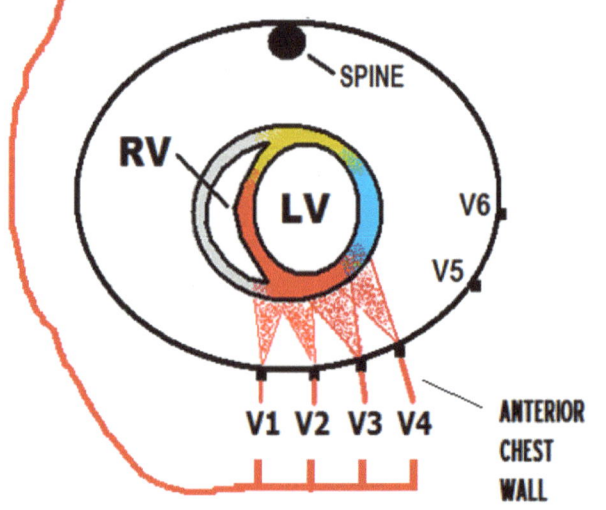

When Anterior Wall STEMI presents WITHOUT ST Elevation in Leads I and AVL or reciprocal ST Depression in Leads II, III and AVF, it is an indicator that the occlusion is located in the MID- LEFT ANTERIOR DESCENDING (LAD) Artery, DISTAL to the first diagonal branch.

ECG presentation consistent with:

ANTERIOR - SEPTAL WALL MI
secondary to obstruction of the Mid- Left Anterior Descending Artery (LAD).

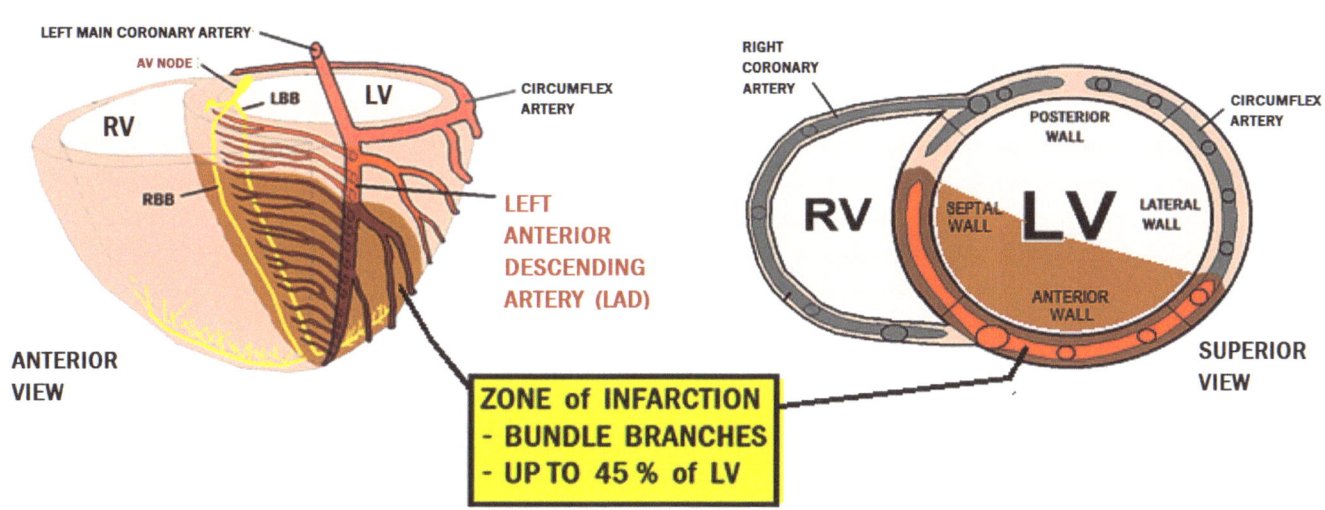

ZONE of INFARCTION
- BUNDLE BRANCHES
- UP TO 45 % of LV

ANTICIPATED COMPLICATIONS of ANTERIOR-SEPTAL WALL STEMI & POSSIBLE INDICATED INTERVENTIONS:	
- CARDIAC ARREST	BCLS / ACLS
- CARDIAC DYSRHYTHMIAS (VT / VF)	ACLS (antiarrhythmics)
- PUMP FAILURE with CARDIOGENIC SHOCK	INOTROPE THERAPY: -DOPAMINE / DOBUTAMINE / LEVOPHED - INTRA-AORTIC BALLOON PUMP (use caution with fluid challenges due to PULMONARY EDEMA)
- PULMONARY EDEMA	- CPAP - ET INTUBATION (use caution with dieuretics due to pump failure and hypotension)
- 3rd DEGREE HEART BLOCK - NOT RESPONSIVE TO ATROPINE	TRANSCUTANEOUS or TRANSVENOUS PACING

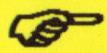 *Scroll through pages in this section to find the 12 Lead ECG with ST PATTERNS which most closely resemble that of your patient's ECG*

☑ **ST ELEVATION Leads V1 – V4, possibly V5, V6**
☑ **ST ELEVATION Leads I & AVL**
☑ **ST DEPRESSION Leads II, III**

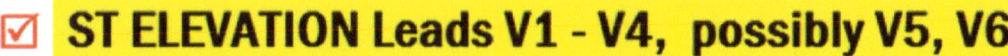

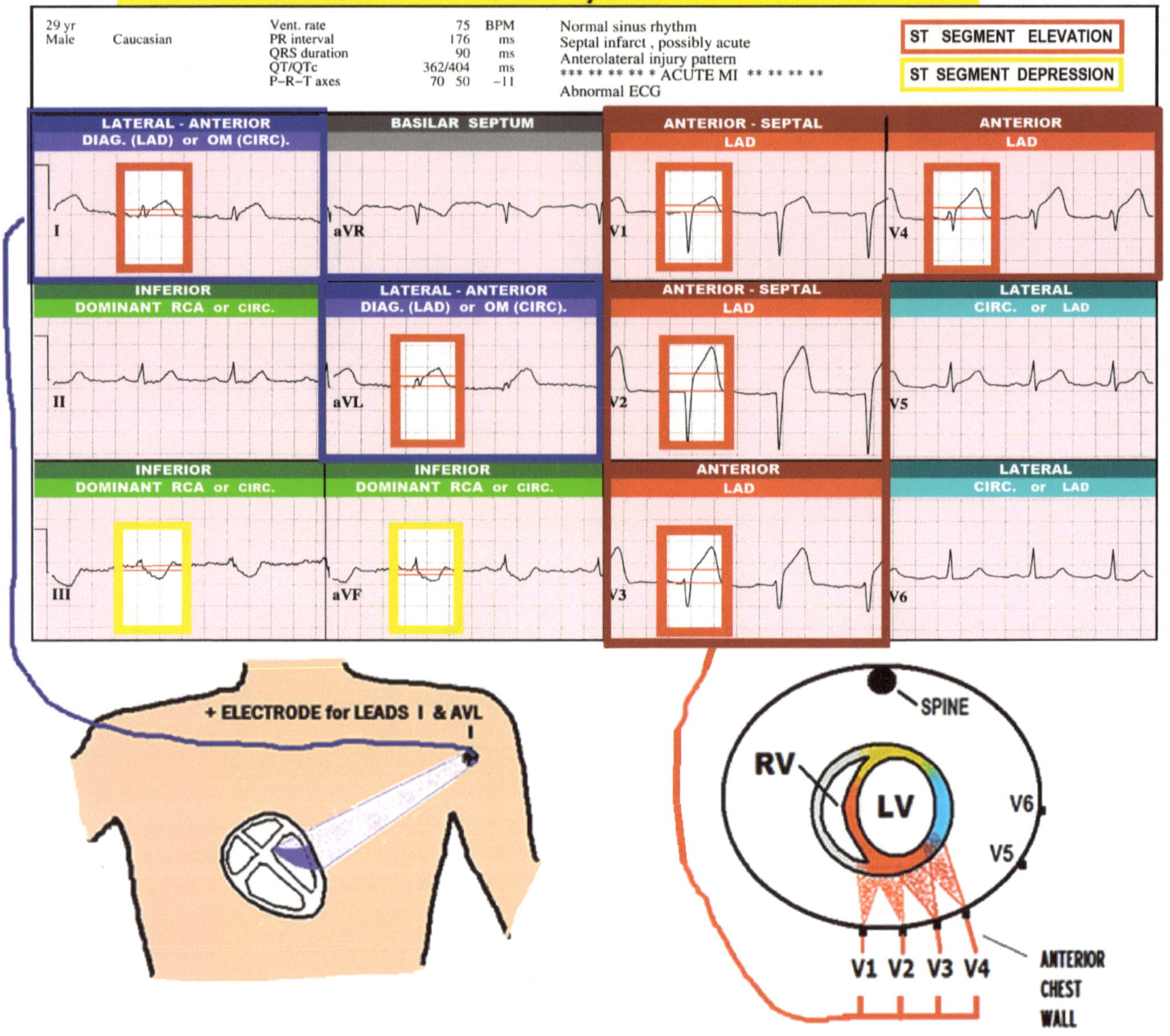

Leads I and AVL view the
ANTERIOR - LATERAL JUNCTION
of the **LEFT VENTRICLE**

Leads V1 – V4 view the
ANTERIOR WALL of the
LEFT VENTRICLE

When ANTERIOR WALL STEMI presents with ST Elevation in Leads I and AVL and reciprocal ST Depression in Leads II, III and AVF, it is an indicator that the occlusion is located in the LEFT ANTERIOR DESCENDING (LAD) Artery PROXIMAL to the first diagonal branch. The zone of infarction is significantly larger than in patients with Anterior Wall STEMI secondary to MID LAD occlusion (as seen in previous example).

ECG presentation consistent with:

ANTERIOR - SEPTAL WALL MI
secondary to obstruction of the PROXIMAL - Left Anterior Descending (LAD) Artery:

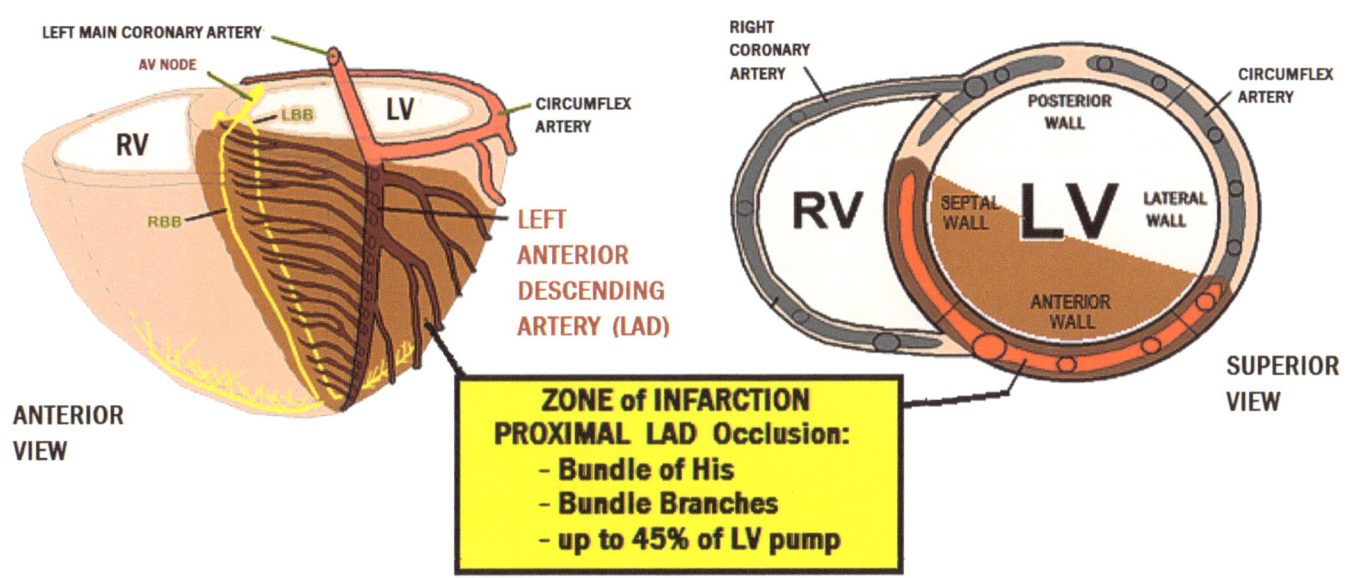

ZONE of INFARCTION
PROXIMAL LAD Occlusion:
- Bundle of His
- Bundle Branches
- up to 45% of LV pump

ANTICIPATED COMPLICATIONS of ANTERIOR-SEPTAL WALL STEMI & POSSIBLE INDICATED INTERVENTIONS:	
- CARDIAC ARREST	BCLS / ACLS
- CARDIAC DYSRHYTHMIAS (VT / VF)	ACLS (antiarrhythmics)
- PUMP FAILURE and CARDIOGENIC SHOCK	INOTROPE THERAPY: -DOPAMINE / LEVOPHED / DOBUTAMINE - INTRA-AORTIC BALLOON PUMP (use caution with fluid challenges due to PULMONARY EDEMA)
- PULMONARY EDEMA	- CPAP - ET INTUBATION (use caution with dieuretics due to pump failure and hypotension)
- 3rd DEGREE HEART BLOCK - NOT RESPONSIVE TO ATROPINE	- TRANSCUTANEOUS or TRANSVENOUS PACING

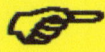 *Scroll through pages in this section to find the 12 Lead ECG with ST PATTERNS which most closely resemble that of your patient's ECG*

☑ **ST ELEVATION LEADS II, III, and AVF**

☑ **Possible SLIGHT ST Elev V5, V6**

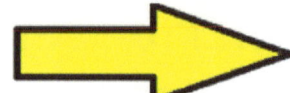 **NO ST Elevation in Lead I or AVL !!**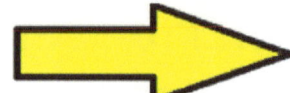

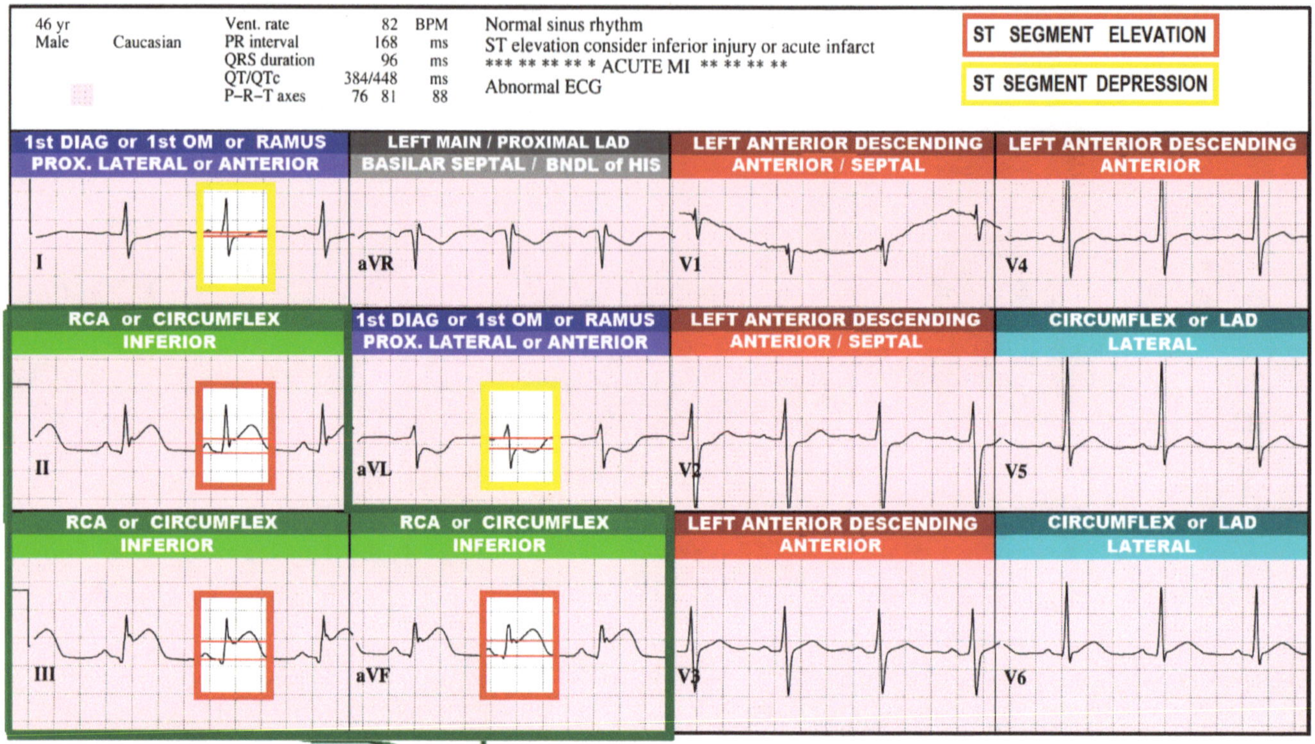

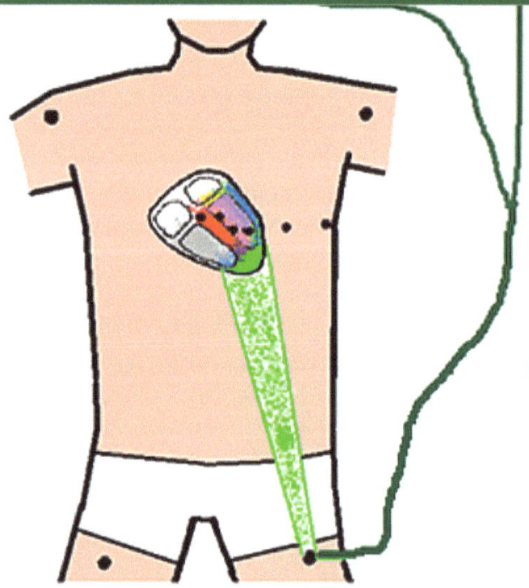

| 46 yr Male | Caucasian | Vent. rate 82 BPM
PR interval 168 ms
QRS duration 96 ms
QT/QTc 384/448 ms
P–R–T axes 76 81 88 | Normal sinus rhythm
ST elevation consider inferior injury or acute infarct
********** ACUTE MI **********
Abnormal ECG | ST SEGMENT ELEVATION
ST SEGMENT DEPRESSION |

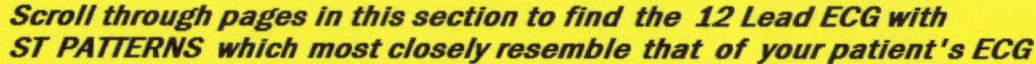

Leads II, III & AVF view the INFERIOR WALL

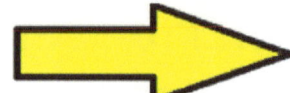 **In cases of INFERIOR WALL STEMI, obtain a RIGHT SIDED ECG to rule out RIGHT VENTRICULAR MI BEFORE giving NITRATES or DIURETICS**

(RCA) in 75-80% of the Population, and from the CIRCUMFLEX ARTERY in 10-15% of the Population. Since the RCA feeds the INFERIOR WALL in 75-80% of the patient population -- and it also feeds the RIGHT VENTRICLE -- we must RULE OUT RIGHT VENTRICULAR MI BEFORE any NITRATES or DIURETICS are given. The 12 LEAD ECG DOES NOT VIEW THE RIGHT VENTRICLE; to rule out RV MI, a RIGHT SIDED ECG must be obtained (see page 7 for more information).

ECG presentation consistent with:

INFERIOR WALL MI
secondary to occlusion of a dominant Right Coronary Artery (RCA).

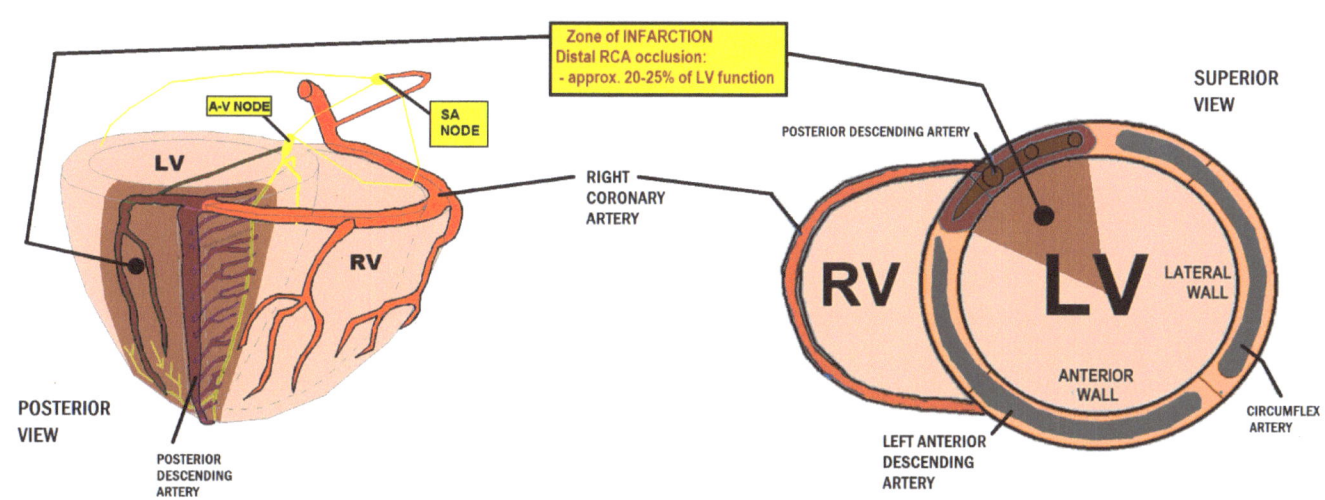

ANTICIPATED COMPLICATIONS of INFERIOR WALL STEMI secondary to RCA Occlusion & POSSIBLE INDICATED INTERVENTIONS:	
- CARDIAC ARREST	BCLS / ACLS
- CARDIAC DYSRHYTHMIAS (VT / VF)	ACLS (antiarrhythmics)
- SINUS BRADYCARDIA	ATROPINE 0.5mg, REPEAT as needed UP TO 3mg. (follow ACLS and/or UNIT protocols)
- HEART BLOCKS (1st, 2nd & 3rd Degree HB)	ATROPINE 0.5mg, REPEAT as needed UP TO 3mg, Transcutaneous Pacing, (follow ACLS and/or UNIT protocols)
- RIGHT VENTRICULAR MYOCARDIAL INFARCTION	- The standard 12 Lead ECG does NOT view the Right Ventricle. - You must do a RIGHT-SIDED ECG to see if RV MI is present. - Do NOT give any Inferior Wall STEMI patient NITRATES or DIURETICS until RV MI has been RULED OUT. (SEE Page 31 for RV MI Interventions)
- POSTERIOR WALL INFARCTION	- POSTERIOR WALL MI presents on the 12 Lead ECG as ST DEPRESSION in Leads V1 - V3. - POSTERIOR WALL MI is NOT PRESENT ON THIS ECG.

☞ *Scroll through pages in this section to find the 12 Lead ECG with ST PATTERNS which most closely resemble that of your patient's ECG*

☑ **ST ELEVATION LEADS - V3R - V6R**
  V LEADS on RIGHT SIDE of CHEST!

☑ **ST ELEVATION LEADS II, III, and AVF**

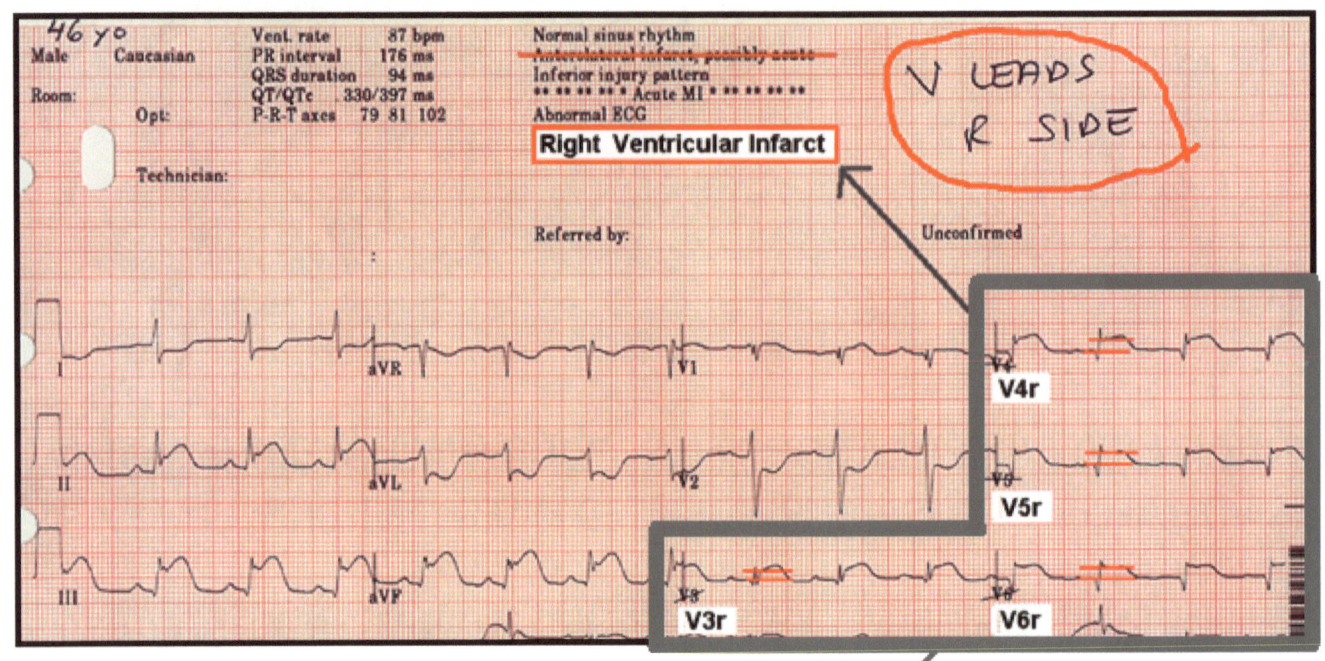

LEADS V3R - V6R VIEW THE RIGHT VENTRICLE

☞ **OBTAIN a RIGHT-SIDED ECG in ALL CASES of INFERIOR WALL STEMI!**

SEE PAGE 7 for more information.

*When a patient with INFERIOR WALL STEMI presents with ST Elevation in Leads I and AVL, it is an indicator that the MI is being caused by a blockage in the proximal aspect of a dominant Circumflex artery, and the patient is most likely suffering from INFERIOR-LATERAL WALL or INFERIOR-POSTERIOR-LATERAL Wall STEMI. Please see pages 32 & 33 for example.

ECG presentation consistent with:

RIGHT VENTRICULAR + INFERIOR WALL MI
secondary to occlusion of a PROXIMAL Right Coronary Artery (RCA).

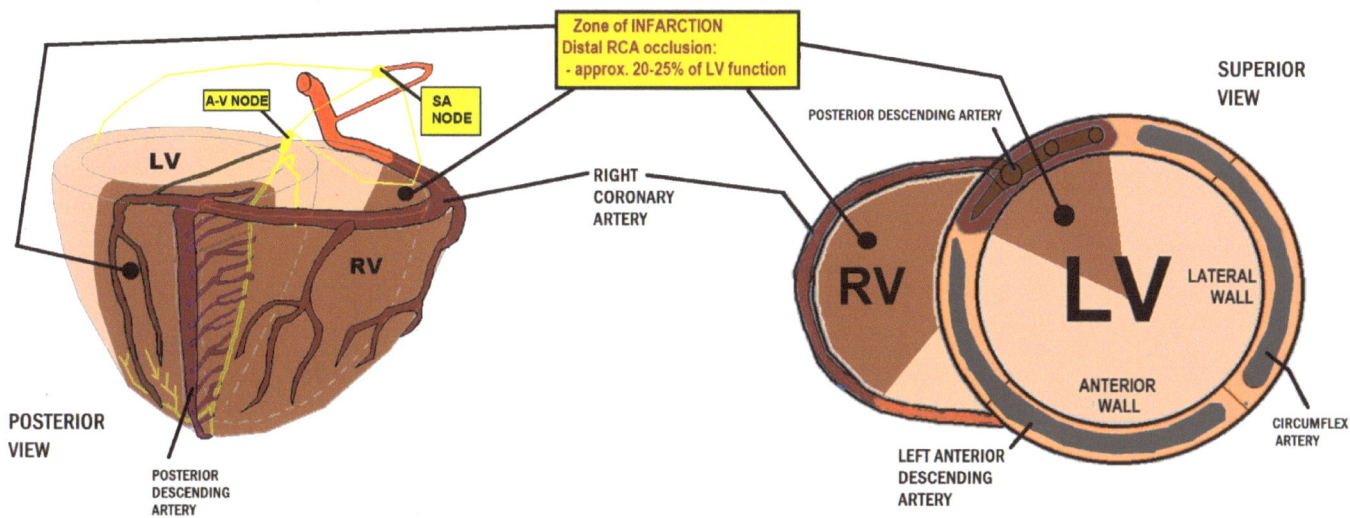

ANTICIPATED COMPLICATIONS of INFERIOR - RIGHT VENRICULAR WALL STEMI secondary to PROXIMAL RCA Occlusion & POSSIBLE INDICATED INTERVENTIONS:	
- CARDIAC ARREST	BCLS / ACLS
- CARDIAC DYSRHYTHMIAS (VT / VF)	ACLS (antiarrhythmics)
- SINUS BRADYCARDIA	ATROPINE 0.5mg, REPEAT as needed UP TO 3mg. (follow ACLS and/or UNIT protocols)
- HEART BLOCKS (1st, 2nd & 3rd Degree HB)	ATROPINE 0.5mg, REPEAT as needed UP TO 3mg, Transcutaneous Pacing, (follow ACLS and/or UNIT protocols)
- RIGHT VENTRICULAR MYOCARDIAL INFARCTION	- NITRATES and DIURETICS are CONTRA-INDICATED. - TREAT HYPOTENSION WITH FLUIDS. (It is Not uncommon to give 500-2000ml of NORMAL SALINE to stabilize BP.
- POSTERIOR WALL INFARCTION	- POSTERIOR WALL MI presents on the 12 Lead ECG as ST DEPRESSION in Leads V1 - V3. - POSTERIOR WALL MI is NOT PRESENT ON THIS ECG.

 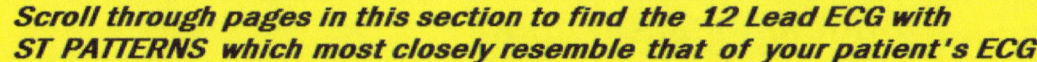

Scroll through pages in this section to find the 12 Lead ECG with ST PATTERNS which most closely resemble that of your patient's ECG

☑ **ST ELEVATION LEADS II, III & AVF (INFERIOR MI)**
☑ **ST DEPRESSION LEADS V1 & V2 (POSTERIOR MI)**
☑ **ST ELEVATION LEADS V5 & V6 (LATERAL MI)**
☑ **ST DEPRESSION LEAD AVR - 1mm or more (favors CX lesion)**

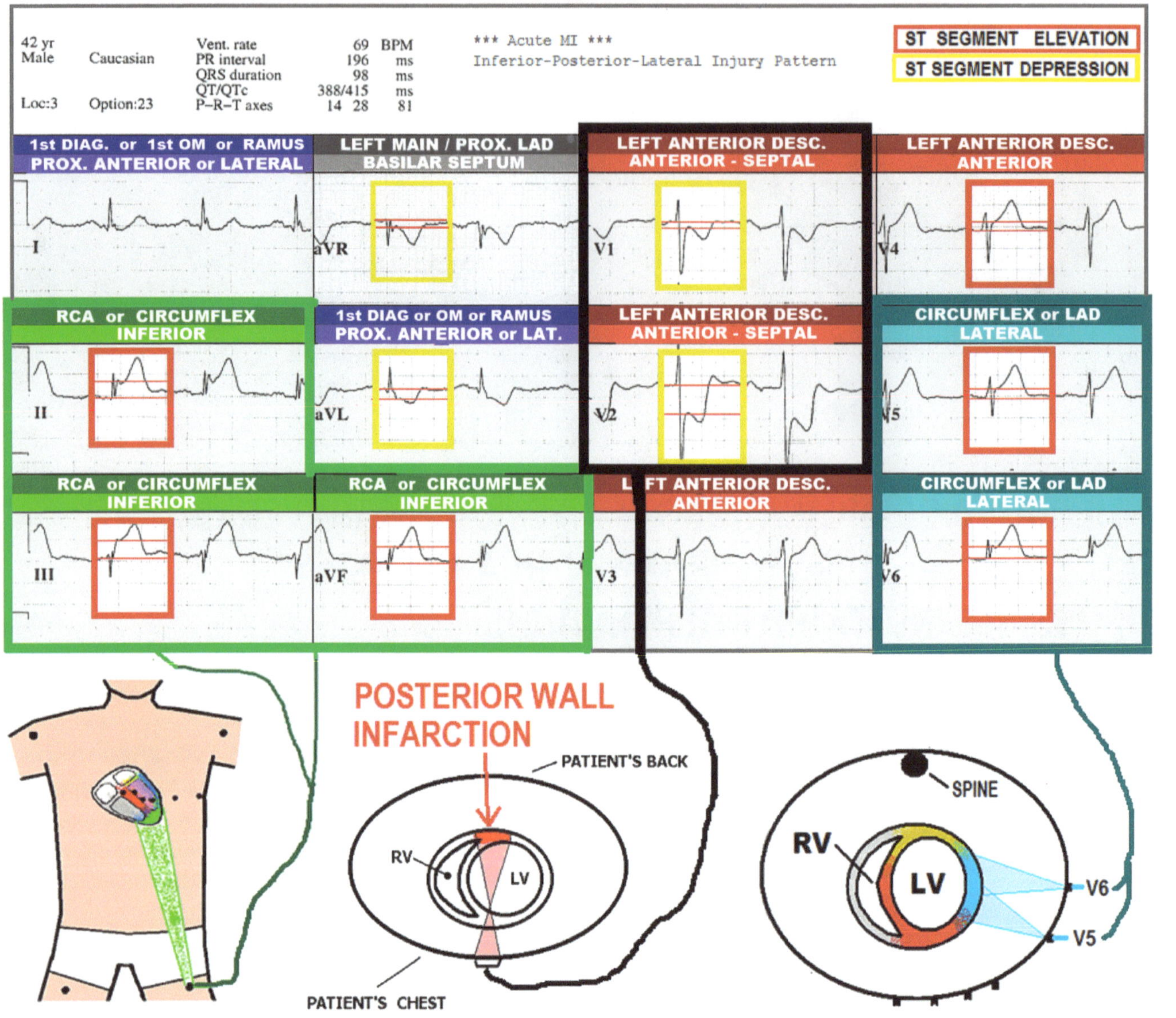

42 yr	Caucasian	Vent. rate	69	BPM	*** Acute MI ***	ST SEGMENT ELEVATION
Male		PR interval	196	ms	Inferior-Posterior-Lateral Injury Pattern	ST SEGMENT DEPRESSION
Loc:3	Option:23	QRS duration	98	ms		
		QT/QTc	388/415	ms		
		P-R-T axes	14 28 81			

1st DIAG. or 1st OM or RAMUS / PROX. ANTERIOR or LATERAL — I
LEFT MAIN / PROX. LAD / BASILAR SEPTUM — aVR
LEFT ANTERIOR DESC. / ANTERIOR - SEPTAL — V1
LEFT ANTERIOR DESC. / ANTERIOR — V4

RCA or CIRCUMFLEX / INFERIOR — II
1st DIAG or OM or RAMUS / PROX. ANTERIOR or LAT. — aVL
LEFT ANTERIOR DESC. / ANTERIOR - SEPTAL — V2
CIRCUMFLEX or LAD / LATERAL — V5

RCA or CIRCUMFLEX / INFERIOR — III
RCA or CIRCUMFLEX / INFERIOR — aVF
LEFT ANTERIOR DESC. / ANTERIOR — V3
CIRCUMFLEX or LAD / LATERAL — V6

POSTERIOR WALL INFARCTION

Figure A   Figure B   Figure C

*Leads II, III and AVF view the INFERIOR WALL, as noted in Figure A; ST elevation in these leads indicates INFERIOR WALL MI (IWMI). In all cases of IWMI, ALWAYS look for Reciprocal ST Depression in leads V1 - V3; it is an indicator of POSTERIOR WALL MI, as shown in Figure B. Posterior MI is seen with both RCA and Circumflex occlusions. Figure C illustrates LATERAL WALL STEMI, as leads V5 and V6 view the LATERAL WALL of the Left Ventricle. During Inferior Wall STEMI when Lead AVR displays ST Depression 1 mm or more, and/or ST Elevation in Lead III > Lead II it is an indicator that the MI results from an occluded Dominant Circumflex Artery, as is the case here; cath lab angiography revealed a 100% obstruction of a dominant circumflex artery, just distal to the 1st obtuse marginal branch. Whenever ST Elevation is noted in Leads I and/or AVL in IWMI, it is a reliable indicator that the blockage is in the proximal aspect of a dominant Circumflex artery, PROXIMAL to the 1st Obtuse Marginal branch (not the case here).

ECG presentation consistent with:

INFERIOR POSTERIOR LATERAL WALL MI
secondary to occlusion of a DOMINANT CIRCUMFLEX Artery (CX).

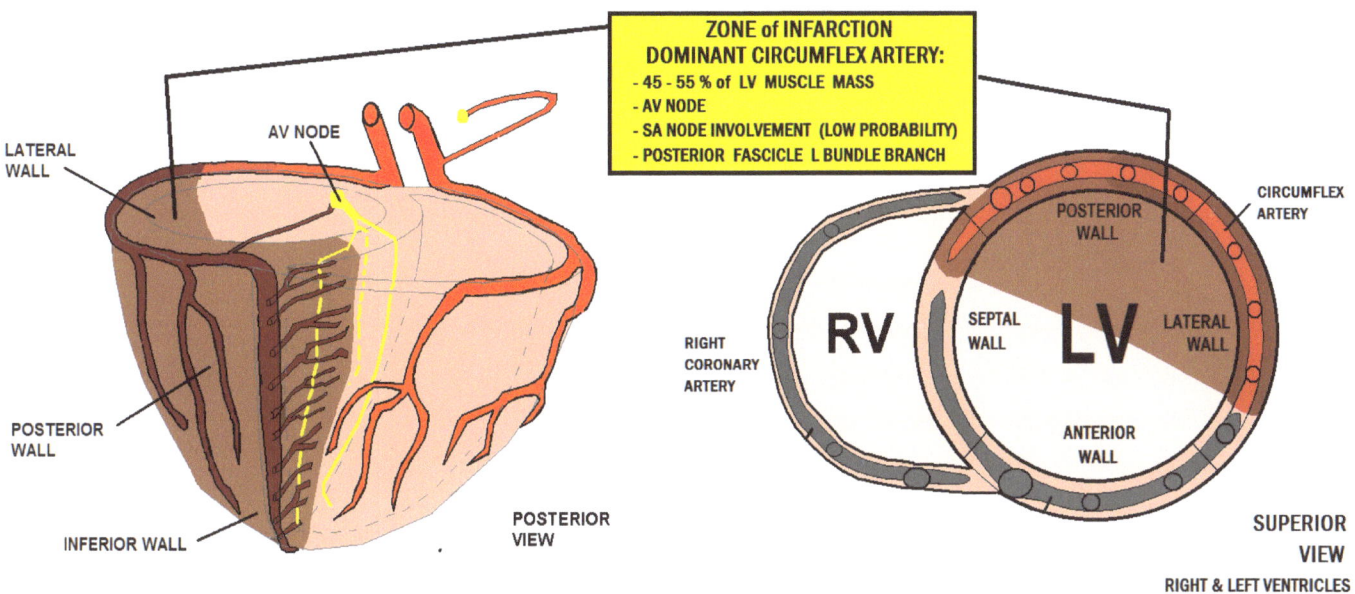

ANTICIPATED COMPLICATIONS of INFERIOR - POSTERIOR - LATERAL WALL STEMI secondary to DOMINANT CIRCUMFLEX ARTERY Occlusion & POSSIBLE INDICATED INTERVENTIONS:	
- CARDIAC ARREST	BCLS / ACLS
- CARDIAC DYSRHYTHMIAS (VT / VF)	ACLS (antiarrhythmics)
- SINUS BRADYCARDIA	ATROPINE 0.5mg, REPEAT as needed UP TO 3mg. (follow ACLS and/or UNIT protocols)
- HEART BLOCKS (1st, 2nd & 3rd Degree HB)	ATROPINE 0.5mg, REPEAT as needed UP TO 3mg, Transcutaneous Pacing, (follow ACLS and/or UNIT protocols)
- CARDIOGENIC SHOCK	- INOTROPE THERAYPY: DOPAMINE 2-10 mcg/kg/min (titrate up to 20 mcg/kg/min). DOBUTAMINE 2-20 mcg/kg/min NOREPINEPHRINE 5-30 mcg/kg/min
- ACUTE MITRAL REGURGITATION	- In cases of inadequate reperfusion, necrosis of Inferior-Posterior-Lateral surfaces may lead to acute papillary muscle tear and Acute Mitral Regurgitation (S1 MURMUR)

☑ **PRIMARY ST ELEVATION in LEADS I & AVL**
☑ **Possible ST Depression Leads II, III, & AVF**

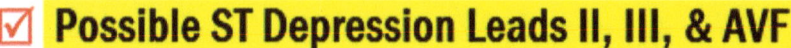

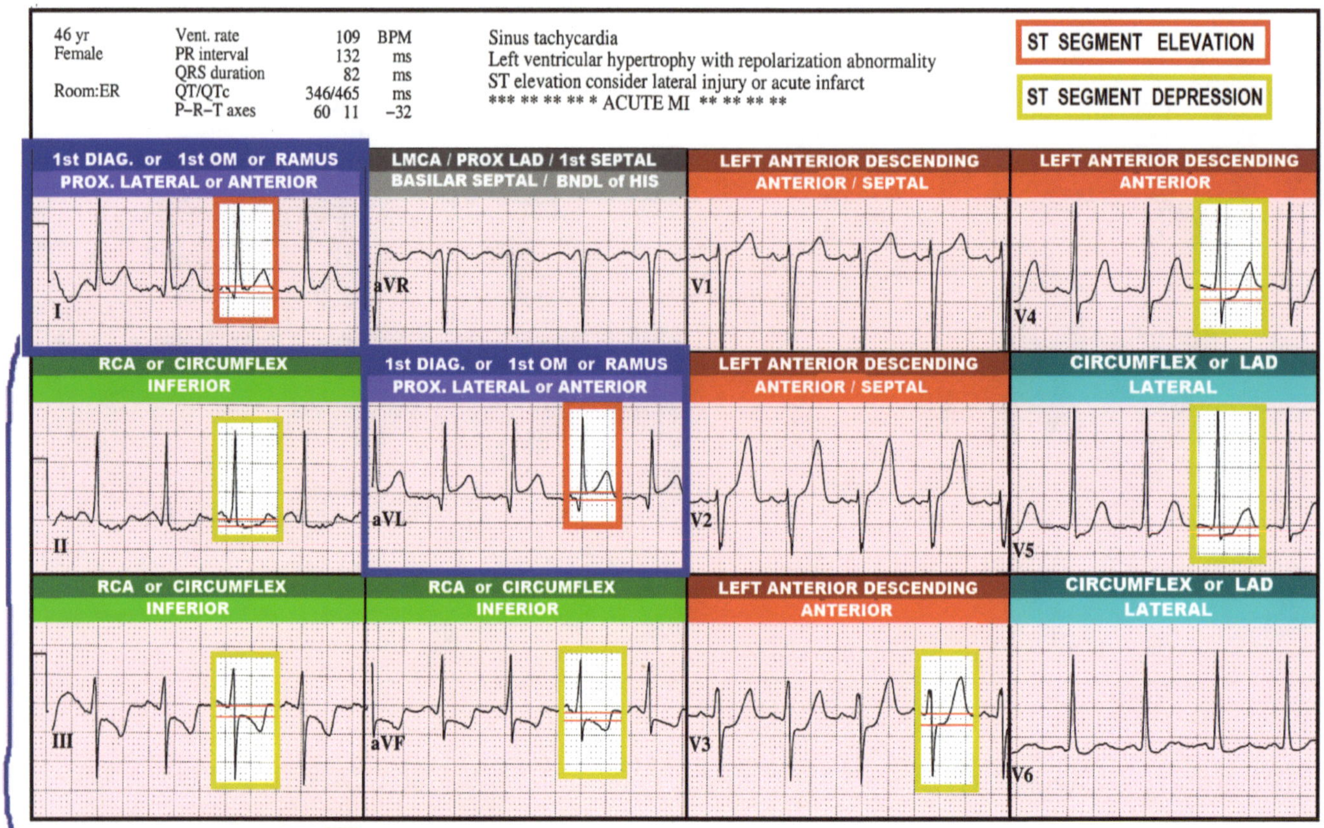

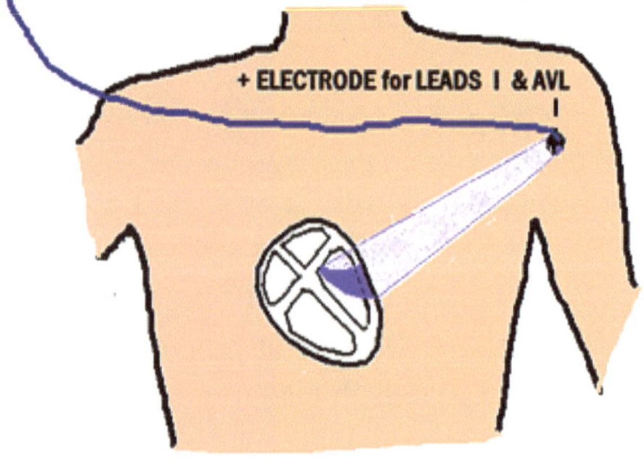

Leads I and AVL view the PROXIMAL aspects of the ANTERIOR and LATERAL Left Ventricle.

*When ST Elevation noted only in Leads I and AVL, it's indicative of an obstruction in the 1st Diagonal Artery (first side-branch of the LAD, supplies upper Anterior Wall or the 1st Obtuse Marginal Artery (first side-branch of the Circumflex Artery that supplies the Lateral Wall). When ST Elevation is noted in Anterior Leads V1-V4 combined with Leads I and AVL, it's indicative of obstruction of the LAD, PROXIMAL to the FIRST DIAGONAL Side-branch -- in other words, a massive MI involving ALL of the ANTERIOR WALL (see pages 26 & 27 for example). When ST Elevation is noted in LEAD AVR, the obstruction is most likely in the LEFT MAIN CORONARY ARTERY and the infarction zone is global, involving most of the Left Ventricle (see pages 18 & 19 for example). When ST Elevation is noted primarily in Leads V5 and V6 combined with Leads I and AVL, the obstruction is in the PROXIMAL Circumflex Artery (and includes the 1st Obtuse Marginal Artery).

ECG presentation consistent with:

LATERAL WALL MI secondary to obstruction of one of the following:

- RAMUS ARTERY
- 1st DIAGONAL ARTERY
- 1st OBTUSE MARGINAL ARTERY

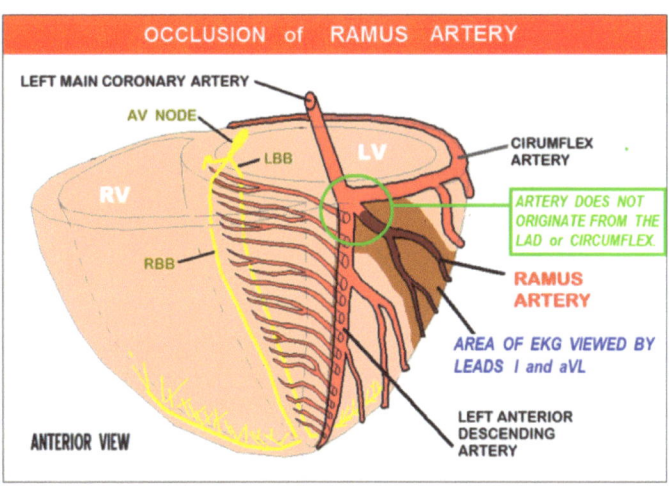

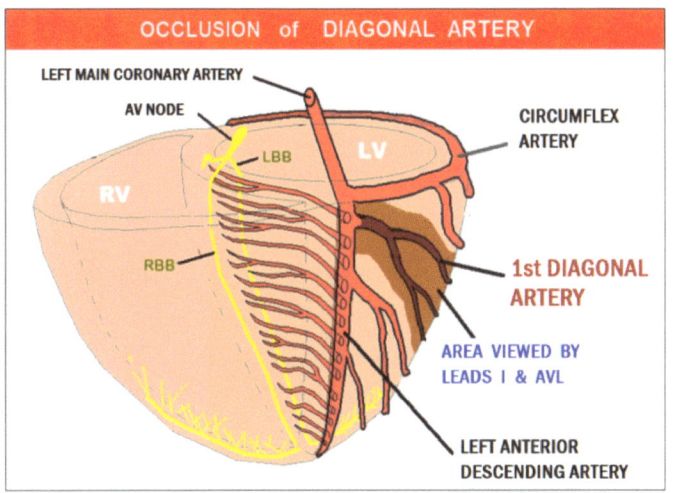

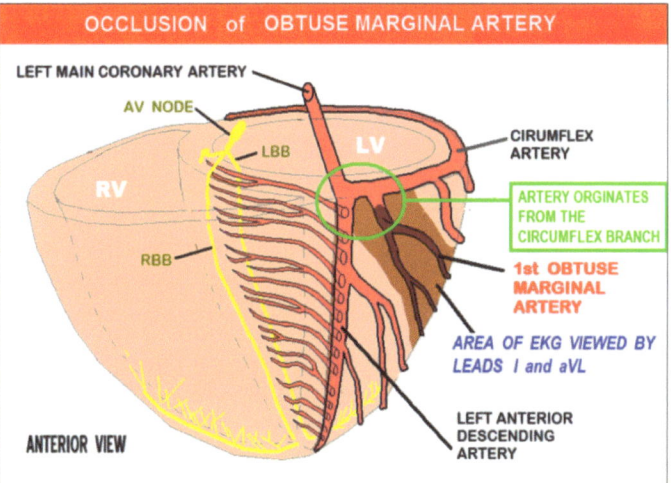

ANTICIPATED COMPLICATIONS of - LATERAL WALL STEMI secondary to Occlusion of RAMUS or Side-branch Artery (1st Diagonal or 1st Obtuse Marginal) and possible interventions to consider:	
CARDIAC ARREST	BCLS and ACLS
DYSRHYTHMIAS	ACLS
- MILD HYPOTENSION	- FLUID CHALLENGE(S): Small fluid bolus, 200-300ml Normal Saline: Auscultate lungs prior to any fluid bolus(es) to RULE OUT Pulmonary Edema. Re-evaluate patient and repeat as needed
- MODERATE to SEVERE HYPOTENSION	- INOTROPE THERAYPY: DOPAMINE 2-10 mcg/kg/min (titrate up to 20 mcg/kg/min). DOBUTAMINE 2-20 mcg/kg/min NOREPINEPHRINE 5-30 mcg/kg/min

SUMMARY OF ACUTE CORONARY SYNDROMES & CORONARY ARTERY DISEASE

CLASSIFICATION	CONDITION	SYMPTOMS	ECG	LABS
ACUTE CORONARY SYNDROME	**STEMI** S-T SEGMENT ELEVATION MI	• ACUTE CORONARY SYNDROME (ACS) SYMPTOMS ARE PRESENT • ONSET OF SYMPTOMS DURING REST or EXERTION • SYMPTOMS NOT EFFECTED BY POSITION, MOVEMENT or RESPIRATION • SYMPTOMS NOT RELIEVED BY REST or NITRATES	• S-T SEGMENT ELEVATION IN 2 or more CONTIGUOUS LEADS • RECIPROCAL S-T DEPRESSION MAY or MAY NOT BE PRESENT	POSITIVE TROPONIN

	NSTEMI NON-S-T SEGMENT ELEVATION MI		• ECG FINDINGS MAY BE CONSTANT, or INTERMITTENT (with symptoms):
			  ■ ISCHEMIC PATTERNS: S-T SEGMENT DEPRESSION and/or INVERTED T WAVES, or OTHER ISCHEMIC PATTERNS (SEE DIAGRAM, PAGE 115)
			  ■ HYPERACUTE T WAVES
				POSITIVE TROPONIN

	UNSTABLE ANGINA	• NEW ONSET OF CARDIAC CHEST PAIN / ACS SYMPTOMS, or • ONSET OF CARDIAC CHEST PAIN / ACS SYMPTOMS WHILE AT REST, or • CHANGE IN PATTERN OF PREVIOUSLY STABLE ANGINA	• IF S-T ELEVATION IS PRESENT, IT SHOULD SUBSIDE WITH REST (PRINZMETAL'S ANGINA) • ECG MAY BE NORMAL	TROPONIN NEGATIVE or BORDERLINE
NON-ACUTE CORONARY ARTERY DISEASE	STABLE ANGINA	PATIENT HAS EXERTIONAL CHEST PAIN, WHICH SUBSIDES WITH REST and/or REST AND NITRATES. SYMPTOMS ARE PREDICTABLE and FOLLOW A "USUAL PATTERN"		TROPONIN NORMAL
	ASYMPTOMATIC CORONARY ARTERY DISEASE	NONE. THE PATIENT MAY HAVE NOTHING MORE THAN "POSITIVE" RISK FACTORS	• PATTERNS OF ISCHEMIA MAY BE PRESENT, or • ECG MAY BE NORMAL	CRP and/or CHOLEST. MAY BE ELEVATED

LIST OF ABBREVIATIONS and ACRONYMS:

ACC	American College of Cardiology	LOE	Level of Evidence
ACCF	American College of Cardiology Foundation	LV	Left Ventricle, Left Ventricular
ACLS	Advanced Cardiac Life Support	MACE	Major Adverse Cardiac Event
ACS	Acute Coronary Syndrome	mg	Milligrams
AHA	American Heart Association	mm	Millimeters
CABG	Coronary Artery Bypass Graft	mv	Millivolts
CPAP	Continuous Positive Pressure Airway	NEJM	New England Journal of Medicine
CX	Circumflex Artery	NSTEMI	Non-ST Segment Elev. Myocardial Infarction
CXR	Chest X-Ray	NTG	Nitroglycerin
ECG	Electrocardiogram	PCI	Percutaneous Coronary Intervention
EMS	Emergency Medical Services	RBBB	Right Bundle Branch Block
ER	Emergency Room	RCA	Right Coronary Artery
HB	Heart Block	RIC	Remote Ischemic Conditioning
HEART	History, ECG, Age, Risk Factors, Troponin	RV	Right Ventricle, Right Ventricular
HRS	Heart Rhythm Society	STAT	"Statim," Latin for "immediately"
IABP	Intra-Aortic Balloon Pump	STEMI	ST Segment Elevation Myocardial Infarction
IV	Intravenous	TIMI	Thrombolysis in Myocardial Infarction
KVO	Keep Vein Open	UA	Unstable Angina
LAD	Left Anterior Descending artery	VF	Ventricular Fibrillation
LBBB	Left Bundle Branch Block	VT	Ventricular Tachycardia
LMCA	Left Main Coronary Artery		

REFERENCES:

1. Amsterdam EA, et al. 2014 AHA/ACC/NSTE-ACS Guideline
2. O'Gara et al. 2013 ACCF/AHA STEMI Guideline
3. The Joint Commission 2015 National Patient Safety Goals
4. Rautaharju et al. 2009 AHA/ACCF/HRS Recommendations for Standardization and Interpretation of the ECG: Part IV: The ST Segment, T and U Waves, and QT Interval
5. O'Connor et al. Acute Coronary Syndromes: 2010 AHA Guidelines
6. Wagner, GS et al. 2009 AHA/ACCF/HRS Recommendations for Standardization and Interpretation of the ECG: Part VI: Acute Ischemia/Infarction
7. Mahler et al. Circulation Outcomes 2015 The HEART Pathway – Randomized Trial
8. Backus BE, Six AJ et al. Crit Path Cardiol 2010 Chest Pain in the ER: Validation of HEART Score
9. Backus BE, Six AJ et al. Int J Cardiol 2013 Prospective Validation of HEART Score in Emerg Dept
10. Canto, JG et al. JAMA 2000; 283: Clinical Characteristics and Mortality of Patients With AMI Presenting Without Chest Pain
11. MacDonald et al. Emerg Med J 2014 Modified TIMI Cannot be Used to ID Low Risk CP in Emerg Dept
12. Zimetbaum et al. 2003 NEJM The Electrocardiogram in Acute Myocardial Infarctioni
13. Tierala et al, 2009 Journal of Electrocardiollogy; Predicting Culprit Artery in STEMI and Correlation with Coronary Anatomy
14. Wellens HJ Europace 2009 The ECG in Localizing Culprit Lesion in Acute Inferior MI
15. Zimetbaum et al, New England Journal of Medicine 2003; ECG Identification of the Infarct Related Artery
16. Kahled Mahmoud et al. 2013 Egypt Heart J Significance of Dev of AVR in Inf MI
17. Goldberger et al. 2015 Am J Cardiol The Electrocardiogram in Diagnosis of Myocardial Ischemia / Infarction
18. Heusch et al. JACC 2015 Remote Ischemic Conditioning
19. Tamura A World J Cardiol 2014 Significance of Lead AVR in Acute Coronary Syndrome
20. Mehta, S et al NEJM 2010;363:930-42 Dose Comparisons of Clopidogrel and Aspirin in Acute Coronary Syndromes
21. Ruppert W TriGen 2010 "12 Lead ECG Interpretation in ACS with Case Studies from the Cardiac Cath Lab"

About the Author and Editorial Board:

Wayne W. Ruppert, CVT, CCCC, NREMT-P is an Interventional Cardiovascular and Electrophysiology Technologist who has logged over 13,000 cardiac catheterizations and electrophysiology studies during the past 20 years. He is certified as a Cardiovascular Clinical Coordinator by the Society of Cardiovascular Patient Care and has coordinated the successful Chest Pain Center and Atrial Fibrillation Center accreditation of Bayfront Health Dade City in Dade City, Florida. In 2010 he authored "12 Lead ECG Interpretation in Acute Coronary Syndrome with Case Studies from the Cardiac Catheterization Lab," a 304 page textbook that is marketed and distributed worldwide by the Ingram Book Company. Mr. Ruppert is a frequent presenter at medical conferences and workshops nationwide. Between 1980 and 1994 he served as a Paramedic, Firefighter, Field Training Officer, Education and QI Director. He currently serves as the Cardiovascular Clinical Coordinator for Bayfront Health Dade City in Florida.

Barbara E Backus, MD, PhD of the University Medical Center Ultrecht, Department of Cardiology, Utrecht, Netherlands. Dr. Backus is the developer of the HEART Score, and has reviewed and edited the Risk Stratification section of this book (pages 15 & 16). To date, Dr. Backus has authored 24 academic journal articles. Her areas of expertise include Research, Emergency Medicine and Cardiology.

Anna Ek, BSN, RN is an Accreditation Review Specialist for the Society of Cardiovascular Patient Care. Anna Ek joined the Society with a strong background in cardiac, surgical, and PACU nursing. She began her nursing career during the time of thrombolytic trials which ignited her longtime passion for cardiology. She has a strong interest in EMS practices and has met with EMS throughout the United States. She is a strong advocate of EMS and the part they play in the pre-hospital care of the cardiac patient. In addition, Anna has a keen interest in induced hypothermia therapy and is working with the Society to research its effects on the post-cardiac arrest patient.

Michael R Gunderson is the American Heart Association's National Director for Clinical Systems in the Quality and Health Information Technology. He has served in emergency healthcare for over 40 years in various leadership, managerial and clinical roles. Among his previous positions, Mic served as the Executive Director for the Kent County EMS System in Grand Rapids, MI.; President of Integral Performance Solutions (IPS); National Director for Quality, Education and Research with the Rural/Metro Corporation; Director of Research and Education with the Office of the Medical Director in the Pinellas County, Florida EMS system; and as a Research Associate in the Department of Surgery at the University of South Florida College of Medicine where he was engaged in studies of oxygen transport physiology, shock and resuscitation. Mic has also served as a field EMT, paramedic and firefighter with military, private and governmental EMS agencies.

William Parker, PharmD, CGP is the Director of Pharmacy Services for Bayfront Health Dade City, Dade City Florida. He is a Registered Consultant Pharmacist and a Board Certified Geriatric Pharmacist. Will is experienced in the evaluation and implementation of Clinical Pharmacy Programs. He received his Bachelor of Science degree in Biomedical Sciences from the University of South Florida and his Doctoral of Pharmacy degree from the University of Florida.

"12 Lead ECG Interpretation in Acute Coronary Syndrome with Case Studies from the Cardiac Catheterization Lab"
This 304 page color textbook features detailed descriptions of typical and atypical coronary artery anatomy and features dozens of case studies which correlate 12 Lead ECG findings with coronary arterial angiography and physiologic changes which occur during cases of ST Segment Elevation Myocardial Infarction (STEMI), Non-STEMI and Unstable Angina.

Book information: www.TriGenPress.com. Select: Booklist
TriGen Publishing 2010
Marketed and Distributed worldwide by the Ingram Book Company

STEMI Assistant tutorial video(s): www.ECGtraining.org→ STEMI Assistant → Tutorial Videos

APPENDIX:

STEMI ALERT - PRIMARY PCI PATIENT: Physician Orders

STEMI Alert declared at _____ hours due to ECG findings consistent with STEMI

Page 1 of 2

Date/Time: _____/_____/_____ at: _____ hours

Pre-checked ☑ orders have been selected based on current evidence-based medicine, and are consistent with current AHA/ACC 2013 guidelines for STEMI. Bulleted (●) orders indicate standard hospital procedures. To DESELECT any of these orders, draw a line through the entire order and initial it.

ALLERGIES: _____

WEIGHT: _____ lbs / kg (circle one)   HEIGHT: _____ (ft/in)

THESE ORDERS EXPIRE IMMEDIATELY AFTER COMPLETION OF CARDIAC CATHETERIZATION

INTERVENTIONAL CARDIOLOGIST: _____

ADMITTING PHYSICIAN: _____

DIAGNOSIS: STEMI

CONDITION: CRITICAL

_____

NURSING ORDERS:

- ● Position CRASH CART in close proximity to patient.
- ☑ If INFERIOR WALL MI is noted on current 12 Lead ECG, obtain tracing of Lead V4R.
- ☑ **ACLS PROTOCOLS for DYSRHYTHMIA MANAGEMENT**
- ● If patient outside of ER, page RAPID RESPONSE TEAM STAT
- ☑ NOFITY the ON-CALL **Interventional Cardiologist** for STEMI ALERT -- STAT.   Time notified:_____
- ☑ NOFITY the ON-CALL Cardiac Cath Lab Call Team for STEMI ALERT -- STAT.   Time notified:_____
- ● Continuous cardiac monitoring
- ● Initiate I.V. sites x 2; preferably 18g or larger, prefer one in the left AC, Normal Saline to Keep Vein Open
- ● Keep patient NPO except medications
- ● Clip and prep bilateral groins -- DO NOT DELAY above procedures or delay cath lab transport for groin clipping
- ● Obtain informed consent for: Left Heart catheterization including angiography with possible PCI / STENT intervention with possible coronary artery bypass surgery and indicated procedures; Peripheral vascular angiography and/or intervention; Moderate sedation.

LABORATORY:

- ● TROPONIN STAT
- ● CBC STAT (unless obtained and charted within last 24 hours)
- ● CMP STAT (unless obtained and charted within last 24 hours)
- ● PT/PTT/INR STAT (unless obtained and charted within last 24 hours)
- ● DRUG SCREEN STAT (unless obtained and charted within last 24 hours)

Other labs: _____

RADIOLOGY:

- ☐ STAT CXR
- ☑ *DO NOT DELAY TRANSPORT TO THE CATH LAB FOR LAB/RADIOLOGY PROCEDURES / RESULTS!*

PATIENT LABEL:

_____

Physician Signature / date / time

STEMI ALERT - PRIMARY PCI PATIENT: Physician Orders

page 2 of 2

Date/Time: _____

- [x] **DO NOT DELAY TRANSPORT TO THE CATH LAB for ANY MEDICATION ADMINISTRATION** --- except for emergency medications to treat/prevent cardiac arrest and/or lethal dysrhythmias.

MEDICATIONS:

- [x] **Oxygen:** Room air only for patients with SAO2 levels 92 - 100%. If SAO2 <92% and/or symptoms of hypoxemia present, administer O2; titrate to maintain SAO2 92 - 99%

- [x] **Aspirin:** Four 81 mg (324 mg total dose) chewable baby aspirin PO NOW unless contraindicated or already given by EMS/ER/nursing unit. If baby aspirin not available patient is to chew one (Non-enteric coated) 325mg adult strength aspirin PO. (If unable to take PO – 300mg PR suppository.) **(CLASS I, Level of Evidence B)**
  TIME GIVEN: _____ REASON IF WITHHELD: _____

- [x] **Nitroglycerin** 0.4mg sublingual every 5 minutes x 3 doses as needed for chest pain,
  DO NOT ADMINISTER Nitroglycerin if Right Ventricular MI is noted, if systolic BP is less than 90mm/hg and/or if patient has taken: Viagra or Levitra in last 24 hours, or Cialis in last 48 hours.

- [ ] **Nitroglycerin IV Infusion:** Begin at 5-10mcg/minute and titrate up to 100mcg/minute to control angina not relieved by SL NTG. Maintain SBP>=100mmHg.
  DO NOT ADMINISTER Nitroglycerin if Right Ventricular MI is noted, if systolic BP is less than 90mm/hg and/or if patient has taken: Viagra or Levitra in last 24 hours, or Cialis in last 48 hours.

- [x] **Morphine:** 2-5mg IV every 5 - 30 minutes PRN for pain

P2Y12 INHIBITORS   (CLASS I, LEVEL OF EVIDENCE B)

- [ ] **Clopidogrel (Plavix®): 600 mg.** Oral.
- [ ] **Clopidogrel (Plavix®): 300 mg.** Oral.
  DOSE GIVEN: _____ DATE: ___/___/___ AT: _____ hours by: _____

  -- or --

- [ ] **Ticagrelor (Brilinta ®): 180 mg.** Oral
  DOSE GIVEN: _____ DATE: ___/___/___ AT: _____ hours by: _____

ANTICOAGULATION   (May defer to Cardiology - DO NOT DELAY STAT TRANSFER to Cath Lab)

- [ ] **Heparin, Unfractionated   (UFH)**
  - ☐ Heparin bolus: _____ Units/kg IV bolus
  - ☐ Heparin drip: _____ Units/kg/hour IV infusion, titrate to maintain ACT between _____ and _____.
  - ☐ OTHER: _____ Dose: _____ Route of Admin: _____

BETA BLOCKER (May defer to Cardiology - DO NOT DELAY STAT TRANSFER to Cath Lab)

- [ ] Metoprolol 5 mg IV bolus, repeat dose X 2, at two minute invervals, assess patient between doses (15mg max. dose),
  WITHHOLD Metoprolol if any of the CONTRAINDICATIONS listed below are present.
- [ ] Metoprolol _____ mg tablet PO; if IV Metoprolol was given, begin PO dose 15 minutes AFTER last IV dose.
  WITHHOLD Metoprolol if any of the CONTRAINDICATIONS listed below are present.
- [ ] OTHER: _____ Dose: _____ Route of Adm: _____ Frequency: _____

PLEASE NOTE if any of the following CONTRAINDIACATIONS are present, withhold Beta Blocker and notify physician:
- ☐ Symptomatic Bradycardia (HR<60)
- ☐ Active Asthma or Reactive Airway Disease
- ☐ Symptomatic Hypotension (SBP<90)
- ☐ AV Block
- ☐ Moderate / severe LV dysfunction
- ☐ Shock / impaired perfusion

> Use caution when RISK FACTORS for Cardiogenic Shock are noted: age >70, Syst BP <120, Sinus Tach >110 bpm, HR<60 bpm

ADDITIONAL ORDERS:
_____
_____

PATIENT LABEL:

_____
Physician Signature / date / time

www.ingramcontent.com/pod-product-compliance
Lightning Source LLC
Chambersburg PA
CBHW040458240426
43665CB00042B/67